The
Contented
Pregnancy

The Contented Pregnancy

Essential advice from conception to birth

Gina Ford

with Dr Charlotte Chaliha

Vermilion
LONDON

1 3 5 7 9 10 8 6 4 2

Published in 2013 by Vermilion, an imprint of Ebury Publishing

Ebury Publishing is a Random House Group company

The Random House Group Limited Reg. No. 954009
Addresses for companies within the Random House Group can be found at
www.randomhouse.co.uk

A CIP catalogue record for this book is available from the British Library

The Random House Group Limited supports The Forest Stewardship Council® (FSC®),
the leading international forest-certification organisation. Our books carrying the FSC label
are printed on FSC®-certified paper. FSC is the only forest-certification scheme supported
by the leading environmental organisations, including Greenpeace. Our paper procurement
policy can be found at www.randomhouse.co.uk/environment

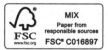

Printed and bound by CPI Group (UK) Ltd, Croydon, CR0 4YY

ISBN 9780091947767

Copies are available at special rates for bulk orders. Contact the sales development team
on 020 7840 8487 for more information.

To buy books by your favourite authors and register for offers, visit
www.randomhouse.co.uk

The information in this book has been compiled by way of general guidance in relation to
the specific subjects addressed, but is not a substitute and not to be relied on for medical,
healthcare, pharmaceutical or other professional advice on specific circumstances and in
specific locations. Please consult your GP before changing, stopping or starting any medical
treatment. So far as the author is aware the information given is correct and up to date as at
March 2013. Practice, laws and regulations all change, and the reader should obtain up to
date professional advice on any such issues. The author and publishers disclaim, as far as the
law allows, any liability arising directly or indirectly from the use, or misuse,
of the information contained in this book.

From Gina
To all the parents who have supported me over the years

From Charlotte
To Maya

Contents

Introduction

If you have picked up this book, you are probably either thinking seriously about becoming pregnant, or are already pregnant. Firstly, congratulations on entering this new stage of your life! This is such an exciting time as you prepare for the new life you'll be bringing into the world.

If it's your first pregnancy, you're likely to feel a little daunted about what to expect over the months ahead. You are probably wondering what will happen to your body and the growing baby inside you, and how you can best prepare for the arrival of the new addition to your family.

My previous books have focused on how to care for your baby, and yourself, after birth, but many mothers have been keen to have more guidance on the stages before the baby is born. My aim in this book is to help support you through your pregnancy. I've teamed up with consultant obstetrician Charlotte Chaliha to provide detailed information on every aspect of pregnancy, so you can feel informed and reassured, and get on with enjoying your pregnancy.

This book covers everything from fertility and conception to birth and the first few weeks with your baby. It will walk you through every month of pregnancy, showing how the embryo develops into a baby and how your body will change. There is lifestyle advice on nutrition and exercise, plus guidance on preparing your nursery and taking care of your relationships as your life changes. You will also learn all about the different options ahead of you for birth and how to draw up your birth plan. The book then provides detailed information on labour and guidance on what to expect in the first few weeks with your baby.

No matter whether this is your first baby or whether you are extending your family, *The Contented Pregnancy* will give you all the tools you need to look forward to the journey ahead.

Good luck! And I hope that your pregnancy is a contented one!

Gina Ford

PART 1

The Pregnancy Basics

1

Fertility and Conception

Whether you're taking the first steps down the road to parenthood, or intending to add to your family, the period between deciding to try for a baby and conception can be an intense one. It can also be a great time to start laying the foundations for a healthy and happy pregnancy.

Some women may fall pregnant at the drop of a hat, but many will find it takes a few months after stopping birth control. Take this opportunity to read up on conception and ovulation, as well as changes you can make to your diet and exercise regime to improve your chances of conception.

If you're already pregnant, then feel free to skip ahead to Chapter 2, although you might be interested to read some of the information below.

Conception basics

Before looking at the steps you can take towards getting pregnant, it's useful to have a basic understanding of conception. Here is a quick low-down on how conception takes place.

● You are born with around one million immature eggs in your body, some of which will be lost by the time you have your first period.

- Every month follicle-stimulating hormone (FSH) is released from your pituitary gland, enabling some of your follicles to ripen. These produce oestrogen, which encourages the uterus to thicken in case a fertilised egg is implanted in it.

- In each cycle 10–20 follicles develop, but only the ripest is released (ovulation).

- The ripe egg travels up the fallopian tube.

- Sperm reach the tube usually between 30 minutes and three hours after you have had sex. Fertilisation of the egg usually occurs in the fallopian tube when the egg meets a sperm.

- The fertilised egg is carried down the fallopian tube to the uterus and reaches the uterine cavity 5–6 days after ovulation.

- The fertilised egg, now grown from a single cell to a cluster called a blastocyst, attaches to the uterine lining and eventually develops into an embryo and then into a foetus.

Getting pregnant

You've chosen to have a baby; now it's time to start trying for one! While each couple's journey towards pregnancy is different, and some will find it easier to get pregnant than others, there are many things you can do to improve your chances of conceiving. Regular, unprotected sex two to three times a week is the first thing to try.

Stopping your contraception

Your contraception has helped you to avoid becoming pregnant. Now you're trying for a baby, it's time to put your contraceptives aside. However, depending on the method that you used, some contraceptives stay in your body for a while after you stop them. Here is a list of contraceptives and what you should expect when you stop using them.

Barrier methods
If you have been using barrier methods of contraception, such as condoms or a diaphragm, this will not affect your fertility and there is no reason not to try to get pregnant straight away.

Combined oral contraceptive pill
If you have been taking the Pill, it may take your body a little while to readjust after you stop taking it and you may be advised to wait for one or two cycles to go by before seriously trying to conceive. You may find you become pregnant as soon as you come off the Pill, but you may also find that it takes a few months for your normal fertility to return. This is quite common and won't have any effect on your pregnancy once you do conceive.

Intrauterine devices
If you have an intrauterine device (IUD) or intrauterine system (IUS, or Mirena), you will need to have this removed in order to try to conceive. Your normal fertility is usually restored as soon as an IUD/IUS has been removed. With an IUS, or hormonal IUD, it can take a few months for your fertility to get back to normal.

Contraceptive implant (Nexplanon)

If you have been taking the long-acting contraceptive implant it can take around six weeks before ovulation occurs after it is removed.

Contraceptive injections (Depo-Provera)

If you have been having contraceptive injections, it can take longer to get pregnant as it takes a while for all traces of the drug to leave your body. Therefore, on average, it can be up to six months following the last injection before your normal fertility is restored.

Sterilisation

If you, or your partner, have been sterilised, it is not always possible to reverse the operation and it may not be funded on the NHS. The reversal of sterilisation can be a difficult operation and it is not always successful. Even when a reversal seems to have worked, women who get pregnant after they have been sterilised are at greater risk of an ectopic pregnancy occurring (see page 181). For men who have had a vasectomy, no more than half of reversal operations are successful. The chances of success may be partly affected by the time that has elapsed since the original operation. If more than three years have elapsed, a vasectomy reversal is less likely to be successful.

Knowing your monthly cycle

Being aware of your monthly cycle will help you to work out when you are most likely to be able to get pregnant. Not all women have a regular 28-day cycle and yours may be longer or shorter than this. Whatever the length of your cycle, your most fertile time will be two weeks, or 14 days, before your period starts and you can count back from this if you have a regular cycle, and if you have intercourse around this time, there will be sperm ready to fertilise the egg as it travels down the fallopian tube towards your womb.

Some women know when they ovulate (or release an egg) because they feel a pain at this time on one side of their abdomen. If you don't feel anything, this doesn't mean that you are not ovulating – the majority of women don't notice it. You may become aware that you produce more cervical mucus at certain times of the month and this coincides with ovulation; the mucus is thick and sticky at the start and end of your cycle, and around the time of ovulation you produce more cervical mucus and it becomes thinner, more transparent and stretchy.

You might already be marking the dates your period begins and ends on a calendar; if not, consider starting now. You can also buy kits that tell you when you are ovulating. You can buy these over the counter from a chemist. Alternatively, if you have a smartphone, you might want to try one of the apps available that calculate when you're ovulating for you.

An irregular cycle

If you have an irregular cycle, it will be harder to work out when you are ovulating, but if you are having intercourse every two or three days you will be covering your most fertile time of the month as sperm can survive in your body for at least a few days.

An exact day?

Some women are very concerned about trying to pinpoint the exact day when they are most fertile but, generally, as long as you are having regular intercourse every two or three days when you are hoping to get pregnant this should be often enough for you to be successful.

When is the best time to get pregnant?

Everyone is slightly different, but the list below may help you understand when is the optimum time for you to try to get pregnant.

- Ovulation may take place 14 days before your period starts. Therefore in a 28-day cycle you will ovulate on day 14. You may ovulate on the same day every month or it may happen on different days if your cycle is irregular.
- During ovulation your cervical fluid will be clear. Try stretching it between your finger and thumb. If it stretches, is clear or semi-clear, this is a good sign.
- While ovulation is happening, your cervix is soft, open, high and wet, like your lips, while at other times it is low and closed, resembling the end of your nose.
- An egg is released from the ovaries once every month and will live for 12–24 hours if it is not fertilised. Oestrogen, follicle-stimulating hormone (FSH) and luteinising hormone influence the development of the follicles in the ovary, from which ovulation takes place. The time (about 10 days) between ovulation to menstruation is known as the 'luteal phase'. The remains of the follicle in the ovary from which the egg is released become the corpus luteum and this produces progesterone to prepare the lining of the womb for implantation of the embryo.
- You may notice mild spotting during ovulation, which is normal. However, if it continues for more than a day, see your GP.

How long does it take to get pregnant?

Each couple is different, so while some women may be lucky enough to get pregnant straight away, or at least very quickly, others may take weeks, or even months, to conceive. Statistics show us that less than one-third of couples get pregnant immediately, so you may have plenty of time to prepare yourself. It's also good to keep in mind that if you are over the age of 35, it usually takes longer to conceive than if you are younger. In general, around 85 per cent of couples take up to one year to get pregnant. By the age of 40 your fertility will decrease by 50 per cent and your risk of pregnancy complication increases. Other problems may also affect you getting pregnant, for example fibroids, endometriosis, tubal infection or scarring from previous surgery.

If you are becoming tense as a result of feeling pressurised to start a baby, try to relax and perhaps even go on a 'conception moon', whereby you and your partner go on a special holiday in order to conceive. You may feel more relaxed away from home and work. If you are at all worried about your or your partner's fertility, seek help and guidance from your GP. They will guide you on when and whether to seek further specialist help such as in vitro fertilisation (IVF).

If you are over the age of 35

These days more women are choosing to put off starting a family until they're older for a variety of reasons – perhaps they want to advance their careers or maybe they haven't met the right person yet. Whatever the reason, choosing to have a baby later in life is, of course, completely valid, but women should also be aware that problems with conception and pregnancy are greatly increased over the age of 35, and this fact should be taken into consideration when making that choice.

While a 35-year-old woman may look and feel young, biological changes within her body means that from this age fewer good quality eggs are left in the 'ovarian reserve', making it harder to conceive. The risk of miscarriage (see page 179) becomes greater over the age of 40, and the likelihood of your child having a chromosomal disorder such as Down's syndrome is also greatly increased.

Of course, there are many benefits to being an older mum: financial security, stable careers and settled relationships, to name just three. As an older woman wanting to get pregnant there will be more obstacles in your way to becoming a mum, but being aware of these will help. Talk to your GP if you have any worries. With luck, you will soon be looking forward to a new and rewarding stage of your life.

Preparing for pregnancy

Once you've made the exciting decision that you'd like to have a baby, you might want to start trying straight away. But now it is the perfect opportunity to take a step back and think about your life and the way you live it. The time between deciding to get pregnant and conceiving is an ideal chance to make sure that you are fully prepared for pregnancy in every way possible by being as fit and healthy as you can be. This will not only increase your chances of getting pregnant, it will also help you to enjoy a healthy pregnancy and to be as fit as you can be for giving birth.

If you know that your diet and exercise regime could be improved there are some simple lifestyle changes you can make that will improve your fertility and your health before you try to get pregnant. For example, eating a really healthy, balanced diet that includes at least five portions of fruit and vegetables a day will help, as will keeping your body toned and fit with regular exercise. If you smoke or drink, might you be able to give these up? Think about these issues seriously, as continuing to smoke and drink can have an adverse effect on your fertility, as well as potentially damaging your unborn baby (see pages 15 and 83).

If you have had some time to prepare yourself, you may find that you are feeling fitter and healthier already and that you feel fully prepared to start the exciting journey ahead. However, many women have unplanned pregnancies or fall pregnant quickly without having time to ensure that they are as fit and healthy as they can be. If you are expecting a baby and haven't had time to make any lifestyle changes yet, there is no need to worry unduly. It is not too late to start taking folic acid (see page 18), to give up smoking and drinking (see page 15) or to follow a healthy diet and exercise regime (see Chapters 3 and 5) once you find out that you are pregnant, but the sooner you do this, the better.

A healthy pre-pregnancy and early-pregnancy diet

To keep healthy while you are trying to conceive and when you are pregnant, it is important to think about what you eat. Your diet should consist of a good balance of protein, fat and carbohydrate (see pages 42–4) and eating regularly is important, too. If your life is hectic and you often eat on the run, perhaps missing regular meals and eating unhealthy snacks, now is the time to be more careful about what you are eating and when.

Your five-a-day

You need to consume at least five portions of fruit and vegetables every day. This can include frozen, canned or dried products as well as fresh fruit and vegetables, though fresh should be your first choice if possible. Do be wary of packaging that states that the food includes 'part of your five-a-day' as this information may be misleading. One of your daily portions can be a glass of fruit or vegetable juice or a smoothie. You should aim to eat two portions of protein every day, which can be fish, meat, eggs or pulses such as beans and lentils. You also need carbohydrates and dairy products such as milk or cheese. When you're trying to get pregnant, it's a good idea to eat foods that are rich in folic acid, such as leafy greens or lentils, and iron, such as red meat, spinach or dried fruits, as these are important in pregnancy (see pages 45 and 46).

Caffeine consumption

There is some conflicting evidence as to whether consuming caffeine can affect your fertility, but, to stay on the safe side, it's a good idea to reduce your caffeine intake when you are trying to get pregnant. Common sources of caffeine are coffee, tea, fizzy drinks and chocolate. Do note that even de-caffeinated coffee and tea include some caffeine so do read the labels!

Things to give up before conception

Smoking

Smoking has a major impact on fertility so it's a very good idea to give this up if you can. Women who smoke tend to have a shorter reproductive life than those who don't; smokers are more likely to have fertility problems and even living with a smoker can reduce your chances of getting pregnant. Men who smoke also have reduced fertility.

If you smoke during pregnancy (and before you are aware that you are pregnant), you reduce the amount of oxygen and nutrients your unborn baby is receiving. Your baby's heart has to beat faster as he tries to get oxygen and he is likely to weigh less when he is born. He will possibly even be born prematurely. Smoking also increases your risk of having a miscarriage and of serious complications during pregnancy. Once your baby is born there is a higher incidence of cot death, of childhood illnesses and even of suffering from learning difficulties.

Giving up smoking sometimes seems impossible, but your GP can offer you the advice and support you need to help you through. Once you know you are pregnant, you may find that you now have the incentive and strength to give up smoking for good. (See also page 83 for more on smoking and pregnancy.)

Alcohol

It's best to avoid drinking alcohol altogether when you are trying to conceive and during pregnancy. Excessive consumption of alcohol and binge drinking can affect your fertility as well as your general health. Once you are pregnant, there is a greater risk of experiencing miscarriage, stillbirth or premature birth if you drink. Babies born to women who drink to excess during pregnancy can suffer from foetal alcohol syndrome, which can lead to poor growth, development problems and facial deformities.

If you find it difficult to avoid drinking alcohol altogether when you are trying to conceive, stick to drinking no more than one to two units of alcohol, no more than once or twice a week. (One unit of alcohol is equivalent to half a pint of beer or lager, a single measure of spirits or about half a glass of wine.) This is unlikely to cause serious problems, but binge drinking and drinking excessive quantities of alcohol really are risky. (See also page 51 for more on alcohol.)

Over-the-counter/prescribed drugs

When you are planning to get pregnant, check with your GP or pharmacist that anything you are taking is safe during early pregnancy as there are some common everyday drugs that can pose risks (see pages 86–8).

Recreational drugs

You should give up taking any recreational drugs when you are planning a pregnancy. Many people assume that drugs such as cannabis are fairly harmless, but they can affect your chances of getting pregnant and your future baby's health.

Anabolic steroids

If your partner takes anabolic steroids, which are popular with some male bodybuilders, it could have an adverse effect on his fertility and this is something you should address when you are planning a pregnancy. The effects of anabolic steroids are generally reversible, although it may take some time for your partner's fertility to return.

Your exercise

Getting plenty of regular exercise will help you to keep fit and healthy in preparation for your pregnancy. If you are already taking daily exercise and are fit, then you should keep this up when you are trying to conceive. If you have let this part of your life slip a little recently or are not keen on exercising, it's important to try to find a physical activity that you enjoy – this way you will be far more likely to get fit and keep it up. Taking a gentle form of exercise on a regular basis, such as swimming, walking or yoga is ideal. (See also Chapter 5.)

Dental health tips

If you are planning to have a baby, pay a visit to your dentist first. If you need any dental work that might require X-rays or an anaesthetic, it's a good idea to get it out of the way before you get pregnant. For more about taking care of your teeth during pregnancy, see page 57.

Supplements for pre-conceptual care

You should be able to get most of the nutrition you need from eating well, but as soon as you decide to get pregnant there are some supplements you should also take to ensure that your baby gets the best possible start in life.

Folic acid

One supplement that it is important to start taking, as soon as you decide you are going to try to have a baby, is folic acid. This helps to prevent neural tube defects, such as spina bifida, in babies. Neural tube defects usually occur in very early pregnancy, when the spinal cord is developing, which is why it is so important that you start taking folic acid as early as you can.

You can buy multi-vitamins containing folic acid, which are designed for women who are pregnant or trying to conceive, and this can be a good way of ensuring you have all the vitamins you need in the run-up to pregnancy. If you are planning to rely on a multi-vitamin supplement, make sure that it has sufficient folic acid for your pre-conceptual needs. It should contain 400 micrograms of folic acid, at least. However, if you have had a previous baby suffering from spina bifida or are taking anti-epileptic drugs, suffer from diabetes, sickle cell disease or thalassaemia you will need to take a higher daily dose of folic acid of 500 micrograms.

Vitamin D

Multi-vitamins designed for pregnant women or those who are trying to conceive usually contain vitamin D, which is also important during pregnancy – it ensures that your bones stay healthy and helps your baby to develop properly. It is quite common for women to be deficient in vitamin D, particularly those with dark skin, who have little exposure to sunlight, or those who are obese. If you are pregnant and at risk of vitamin-D deficiency, you should be taking a supplement of 10 micrograms of vitamin D a day.

Conditions to be aware of before you conceive
Rubella

German measles, or rubella, is a very common childhood illness, which is generally mild, but it can be very dangerous for your growing foetus if you contract it when you are pregnant (see also page 188). Most women are immune to rubella because they have been vaccinated at school as a child, but it may be a good idea to confirm this before you try to get pregnant.

If you can't check your own records, you can have a blood test to check your rubella immunity and if you missed the vaccination or are no longer immune, you can have another jab and wait a few months before trying to conceive. If you find out you are not immune to rubella once you are pregnant, it will then be too late to have the vaccination.

Diabetes

If you suffer from diabetes, talk to your GP before you become pregnant to discuss the particular problems you may encounter (see page 193 for more on this). If you are substantially overweight your GP will probably suggest you try to lose weight before you conceive. You will need to take a higher supplement of folic acid and your GP will be able to advise you about this.

It is important to get your blood sugar levels under control before you try to become pregnant and your GP will advise you about this. If your HbA1c level is high, your GP will probably suggest you try to reduce it before you try to conceive, as this can cause problems for you and your baby.

Obesity

We all know the health risks of being overweight or obese and, unfortunately, if your body mass index (BMI) is over 30 (see page 37), it may be more difficult for you to conceive, and more complications for you and your baby can arise during pregnancy and birth. For this reason, it is usually advised that you try to lose weight before you start trying for a baby. It is not a good idea to go on a diet when you get pregnant, so it is usually advised that women should lose the necessary weight a few months before trying to conceive. Losing weight can be difficult and daunting, so if you are having trouble, discuss weight-loss approaches with your GP, who will be able to offer you help and support.

High blood pressure

If you have high blood pressure, you should talk to your GP about your plans to start a family. If you are taking medication for high blood pressure, it may not be suitable to carry on taking it during pregnancy and you may need to change to a different type of medicine. In addition, you will need careful monitoring during pregnancy to make sure that the blood flow to the foetus and the placenta isn't affected by any drugs you are taking to reduce your blood pressure. Having high blood pressure also increases your risk of getting pre-eclampsia, a potentially serious condition. This means that the team caring for you during your pregnancy will be particularly vigilant about this. (See page 191 for more on high blood pressure and pre-eclampsia.)

Recurrent miscarriage

It's a very sad fact that miscarriage is far more common than many people realise. It is estimated that about one in four pregnancies end in miscarriage, and for women over the age of 40 this figure rises to about half of all pregnancies. Sometimes, when pregnancies are lost very early on, women do not even know for certain that they had been pregnant. For women who have had a positive pregnancy test and then gone on to lose their baby, this is an extremely distressing experience and often it is not possible to determine the reasons for it.

If you've had a miscarriage in the past, you may be worried about becoming pregnant again. It is important to try to remember that most women who have had a miscarriage then go on to have a healthy baby.

If you have experienced more than three miscarriages in a row, this is known as 'recurrent miscarriage'. You will usually only be referred for investigations into the cause of your pregnancy losses if you have experienced recurrent miscarriages. There are many potential causes, such as blood-clotting disorders or chromosomal problems, and some are treatable while others, sadly, are not. However, for more than half of all couples who experience recurrent miscarriage a cause will not be found. There are factors that make recurrent miscarriage more likely: women who are very overweight or underweight or women over the age of 35. Recurrent miscarriage is extremely distressing, but even those who have experienced three miscarriages in a row are more likely to go on to have a successful pregnancy than to have another miscarriage. (For more on miscarriage, see page 179.)

Inherited conditions

It's a good idea to be aware of any family history of conditions that could be inherited – in either your family background or your partner's. Ask on both sides of the family to see whether anyone has any prior knowledge that could be good to know about. It is not necessary for either of you to be affected by the disease – you could merely be an unknowing carrier of it. Even if a close relative has suffered, your baby could be at risk. The best plan is to consult your GP in the first instance – they may refer you for genetic screening and counselling.

The following conditions are all inherited:

- Haemophilia
- Cystic fibrosis
- Muscular dystrophy
- Sickle cell anaemia
- Thalassaemia

Some women have easy pregnancies; others are more difficult. It's impossible to predict which yours will be as every woman – and every pregnancy – is different. However, making some small lifestyle changes, especially focusing on healthy eating and regular exercise, will give you a good foundation for a happy and healthy pregnancy.

Discovering You're Pregnant

The moment you and your partner discover that you are going to be bringing a new life into the world together is one of the biggest and most wonderful events that you can go through together. But whether you have been planning a pregnancy for a while, or whether it's come out of the blue, you're bound to be wondering what the next few months will bring.

The first signs of pregnancy

You may have been wondering whether you are pregnant, but are not sure. Perhaps you just have a strange feeling that you feel 'different' from usual. If this is your first pregnancy, then you will have no previous experience to go on. Here are the most usual signs to look for:

- Late or missed periods.

- Nausea or vomiting, especially in the morning.

- Going to the loo more frequently than usual.

- Feeling more tired than usual.

- Having a strange taste in your mouth.

- Noticing that your nipples are larger and darker than usual and/ or that your breasts are sore and/or swollen.

- Cramping and light spotting.

- Aversion to certain foods and drinks that you used to enjoy (e.g. wine, certain cooking smells, coffee).

- Feeling more emotional and possibly crying more than usual.

- Feeling off-colour, perhaps with headaches.

Pregnancy tests

When you suspect that you might be pregnant, you can buy a home pregnancy test in your local chemist's to check whether you are pregnant or not. These tests are very reliable and you can do one as soon as you realise that your period has not started when it should. These tests work by measuring the level of pregnancy hormones (human chorionic gonadotrophin) in your urine and you usually just have to pee onto a stick. Some tests are more sensitive than others and you need to follow the instructions precisely. It is sometimes possible to be given a negative result when you are actually pregnant if you do the test very early, so if your test is negative and your period still doesn't come, you may need to repeat it a few days later.

GP pregnancy tests
Generally, a home urine test is all that you need to confirm whether you are pregnant or not, but your GP may carry out

another urine pregnancy test or a blood test. This can give a very accurate picture of the level of the pregnancy hormones in your body, and so can give an indication of whether you are expecting a multiple birth or an ectopic pregnancy. Your GP may carry out an internal examination to confirm your pregnancy as the cervix changes colour and becomes softer if you are pregnant.

Calculating your due date

Your GP will be able to work out the approximate date on which your baby is due. They will take the first day of your last period to calculate it, so you will need to keep track of this. However, you may not be able to get an accurate date this way if your cycle is longer or shorter than average – or if you can't remember your exact date.

Based on your last period dates, the estimated date is 40 weeks from the first day of your last period. If your cycle is irregular or you cannot remember your last period date then an early ultrasound scan will be useful to date your pregnancy.

How to estimate your delivery date
Put a ring around the first day of your last period (shown in bold type). The date shown in lighter type below is your baby's due date.

January	1	2	3	4	5	6	7	8	9	10	11	12	13	14
Oct/Nov	8	9	10	11	12	13	14	15	16	17	18	19	20	21
February	1	2	3	4	5	6	7	8	9	10	11	12	13	14
Nov/Dec	8	9	10	11	12	13	14	15	16	17	18	19	20	21
March	1	2	3	4	5	6	7	8	9	10	11	12	13	14
Dec/Jan	6	7	8	9	10	11	12	13	14	15	16	17	18	19
April	1	2	3	4	5	6	7	8	9	10	11	12	13	14
Jan/Feb	6	7	8	9	10	11	12	13	14	15	16	17	18	19
May	1	2	3	4	5	6	7	8	9	10	11	12	13	14
Feb/Mar	5	6	7	8	9	10	11	12	13	14	15	16	17	18
June	1	2	3	4	5	6	7	8	9	10	11	12	13	14
Mar/Apr	8	9	10	11	12	13	14	15	16	17	18	19	20	21
July	1	2	3	4	5	6	7	8	9	10	11	12	13	14
Apr/May	7	8	9	10	11	12	13	14	15	16	17	18	19	20
August	1	2	3	4	5	6	7	8	9	10	11	12	13	14
May/Jun	8	9	10	11	12	13	14	15	16	17	18	19	20	21
September	1	2	3	4	5	6	7	8	9	10	11	12	13	14
Jun/Jul	8	9	10	11	12	13	14	15	16	17	18	19	20	21
October	1	2	3	4	5	6	7	8	9	10	11	12	13	14
Jul/Aug	8	9	10	11	12	13	14	15	16	17	18	19	20	21
November	1	2	3	4	5	6	7	8	9	10	11	12	13	14
Aug/Sep	8	9	10	11	12	13	14	15	16	17	18	19	20	21
December	1	2	3	4	5	6	7	8	9	10	11	12	13	14
Sep/Oct	7	8	9	10	11	12	13	14	15	16	17	18	19	20

15	16	17	18	19	20	21	22	23	24	25	26	27	28	29	30	31
22	23	24	25	26	27	28	29	30	31	1	2	3	4	5	6	7
15	16	17	18	19	20	21	22	23	24	25	26	27	28			
22	23	24	25	26	27	28	29	30	1	2	3	4	5			
15	16	17	18	19	20	21	22	23	24	25	26	27	28	29	30	31
20	21	22	23	24	25	26	27	28	29	30	31	1	2	3	4	5
15	16	17	18	19	20	21	22	23	24	25	26	27	28	29	30	
20	21	22	23	24	25	26	27	28	29	30	31	1	2	3	4	
15	16	17	18	19	20	21	22	23	24	25	26	27	28	29	30	31
19	20	21	22	23	24	25	26	27	28	1	2	3	4	5	6	7
15	16	17	18	19	20	21	22	23	24	25	26	27	28	29	30	
22	23	24	25	26	27	28	29	30	31	1	2	3	4	5	6	
15	16	17	18	19	20	21	22	23	24	25	26	27	28	29	30	31
21	22	23	24	25	26	27	28	29	30	1	2	3	4	5	6	7
15	16	17	18	19	20	21	22	23	24	25	26	27	28	29	30	31
22	23	24	25	26	27	28	29	30	31	1	2	3	4	5	6	7
15	16	17	18	19	20	21	22	23	24	25	26	27	28	29	30	
22	23	24	25	26	27	28	29	30	1	2	3	4	5	6	7	
15	16	17	18	19	20	21	22	23	24	25	26	27	28	29	30	31
22	23	24	25	26	27	28	29	30	31	1	2	3	4	5	6	7
15	16	17	18	19	20	21	22	23	24	25	26	27	28	29	30	
22	23	24	25	26	27	28	29	30	31	1	2	3	4	5	6	
15	16	17	18	19	20	21	22	23	24	25	26	27	28	29	30	31
21	22	23	24	25	26	27	28	29	30	1	2	3	4	5	6	7

Date discrepancies

A 'due date' is not the date on which your baby will definitely be born, but an estimate of the time around which your baby will be born. In fact, fewer than five per cent of babies are actually born on their due date. This is because, although pregnancy is calculated to last around 40 weeks, it is quite normal for your baby to be born within two weeks before or after this.

When to tell other people about your pregnancy

When you find out that you're having a baby, the feelings of elation and joy that follow make it very tempting to share your wonderful news with the entire world. This is understandable, but you may prefer not to tell anyone other than close family members until the three-month 'safe period' is up. The first three months are when most miscarriages occur. Having to share the sorrow of losing a baby, if this should happen, with everyone can only add to your distress, which is why many people decide to wait until the end of the first trimester of pregnancy before they spread the news. Keep in mind that doing this can bring with it a new flush of parent-to-be anxieties, as letting everyone know you are going to becoming parents can suddenly make it feel very 'real'. Be ready for a variety of reactions to your news too. Although most people will be thrilled, you might be surprised or hurt if some people's responses aren't what you expected.

You need to tell your employer that you are pregnant at least 15 weeks before your due date (for more on this, see page 263);

however, if you work night shifts or are in a heavy-lifting job, it is advisable to tell your employer as soon as you find out you are pregnant. Your employer has a duty of care for you and will need to do a risk assessment to reduce any risks to your health and safety. For more information on this topic, see www.hse. gov.uk.

Varying emotions

You may find it hard to believe your positive pregnancy test result at first and it may take a little time to adjust to the news. You may feel a wide variety of emotions at this time and it is common to experience a mixture of joy and anxiety. Starting a family involves a huge change in your life; it can take a while to become adjusted to this and you may find that you are full of uncertainties and concerns. It is not uncommon to wonder whether you have done the right thing or to question whether you are really ready for a baby. You may find that you are anxious about the pregnancy itself and about all the potential problems you could face. However, these mixed emotions are very common during pregnancy, on top of which the hormonal changes in your body will be affecting your emotional responses.

To help you think your feelings through here is a list of some of the issues and emotions that parents-to-be commonly feel in the first weeks of pregnancy. Of course you may be lucky enough not to experience any of these concerns, as every couple's approach to pregnancy is different, but it's important to recognise that if you do, this is entirely natural and is no cause for concern.

Things you and your partner might both be worried about

- Even if your pregnancy was planned and much wanted it is not unusual to feel that everything is happening too quickly. For example, you may have assumed that it was going to take you months to get pregnant and it can be a shock if it happens straight away. You may even feel apprehensive about the permanence of what is happening – this is going to change your life forever.

- Feelings of being overwhelmed by the thought of lifelong responsibility for another human being.

- Fears about how the pregnancy and parenthood will affect your relationship with each other.

- Concerns that your parenting skills won't match up to those of your own parents.

- Fears that you might repeat the same mistakes that you feel your parents made with you.

- Financial concerns about the costs of having a baby, especially if one of you is planning to give up work.

- Fears of miscarriage or the health of the baby.

Things that you might be worried about

- You might worry about how your body is going to change during pregnancy and that this is going to affect how attractive your partner finds you.

- Concerns about how this is going to affect your career and what impact it will have on your identity as a person.

- Fears about the birth itself and how you will cope with it.

Things your partner might be worried about

- That he will come second place to the baby or that you might love him less – that there might be less love to go round.

- That you will have less time for him and that he will miss what you used to have.

- That he will not be able to rise to the occasion and be supportive enough to you during the pregnancy.

- That he will not know how to be a good father when his child arrives.

- That he will not be able to support his growing family financially.

- That your relationship is going to change and that your sex life will be affected by parenthood.

- That he will become an outsider during the pregnancy or be pushed out by more knowledgeable female family and friends – or even by doctors and health professionals.

Surprises and Complications

You may not have been trying for a baby when you find yourself pregnant, or you may find out that you're expecting more than one! What is unsurprising is that you will have all sorts of conflicting feelings during this time.

An unplanned pregnancy

If your pregnancy is unplanned you may need to tell your partner some unexpected news and this can be more difficult if you are not sure how he will feel, or if you are unsure how you feel yourself. Having a baby is a major life-changing event and if you haven't planned for this, you will inevitably feel some doubts and worries about whether you are ready – emotionally and financially. Take some time to think through your concerns and discuss them with your partner as calmly as possible.

Managing by yourself

If you are not in a long-term relationship with the father of your expected baby or if you are planning to bring up your baby as a single parent, you may have concerns about how you will cope by yourself. Pregnancy and bringing up a child is an emotional experience, and going through this without the support of a partner can be a daunting prospect. It will really make a difference if you have an established network of family and friends around you so that you can share any worries or concerns, and it is a good idea to try to make sure you link up with other pregnant women through antenatal and other types of classes for pregnant women, so that you have contact with others who are sharing similar experiences. (See page 126 for more on antenatal classes.)

Expecting twins

If you are pregnant with twins, they will be developing in just the same way as a single baby. Multiple pregnancies are monitored more closely during pregnancy, just to be sure that things are progressing well.

There are different types of twin pregnancies, depending on whether they are the result of two separate eggs being fertilised (dizygotic or non-identical twins) or one egg dividing into two (monozygotic or identical twins). Non-identical twins each have their own placenta, but sometimes identical twins share a placenta and may even be developing in the same sac inside the womb.

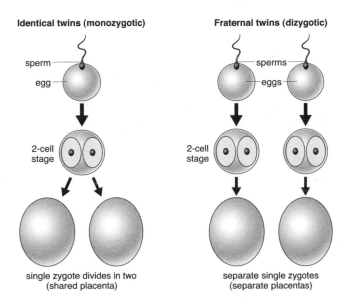

Identical twins (monozygotic)

sperm

egg

2-cell stage

single zygote divides in two (shared placenta)

Fraternal twins (dizygotic)

sperms

eggs

2-cell stage

separate single zygotes (separate placentas)

How identical and non-identical (fraternal) twins are formed

Now that you're pregnant you're likely to feel equal parts exhilarated and terrified. Your life will never be the same again, and that can be quite a daunting thought. If you're feeling anxious at all, talk through your worries with your partner, family, friends, your GP and midwife. You are not alone, and the more you can express your concerns, the easier it will be to conquer them so that you can get extra support if needed.

3
Nutrition During Pregnancy

Eating well in pregnancy is mostly about using your common sense. A healthy diet at this time is very much the same as a healthy diet at any other time; what is good for you is good for your baby and for the pregnancy too. However, with the extra demands pregnancy places on you, both physically and mentally, now is the ideal time to start looking after yourself as well as you possibly can.

Think of eating healthily not as a 'chore' but rather as an opportunity to treat and nurture yourself. Before you were pregnant you might have had that extra glass of wine or treated yourself to a bar of chocolate – without giving it a second thought – but perhaps now is the time to think of alternative ways of rewarding yourself. If you take the time to look after yourself during pregnancy, you will not only be better equipped to deal with the demands of your newborn, but evidence suggests being in optimum health will also help your delivery to go smoothly and ease your recovery post-birth.

Eating well doesn't have to be complicated and it should be enjoyable. During the nine months of pregnancy a good, nutritious diet with a few added extras will benefit both you and your unborn baby, ensuring that he is born at a healthy weight and has all the fuel he needs for developing his brain, skeleton, nervous system and all the other parts that make up his body. You eating a good diet, containing a wide variety of healthy foods, could even affect his taste buds later on in life. Remember: taking care of yourself is taking care of your unborn baby.

Putting on weight in pregnancy

Weight gain in pregnancy can be an emotive issue for many women. You are bound to put on weight as your pregnancy progresses and this is natural and to be expected. Your baby, the placenta and the amniotic fluid weigh a surprising amount, but most of the extra weight disappears quickly after the birth. However, it is common to feel that you might be putting on weight 'in yourself', and you might find this kind of excess weight hard to lose afterwards.

In today's society, in which obesity has reached almost epidemic levels in the population, it is common for women to feel they are being judged as being overweight and you may have learnt to be afraid of gaining. Even if you are really confident about the way you look, you may sometimes feel threatened by images that bombard you daily in newspapers and magazines showing women with so-called 'perfect' bodies – even though it is likely that these have been airbrushed and 'slimmed down'.

There is nothing more natural than gaining weight during pregnancy. It is to be expected and encouraged, but, as with everything in life, it is all about keeping things balanced.

Calorie requirements in pregnancy

We've all heard the old adage about 'eating for two' during pregnancy. The truth is, in pregnancy, our calorific needs don't change from normal that much. The average woman requires roughly 2,000 calories a day and a pregnant woman requires about the same. However, in the third trimester, from the sixth month onwards, the recommendation is that you consume an extra 200 calories a day. That's the equivalent of a slice of cheese on toast, a bowl of cereal or a couple of bananas. In other words, it's not very much.

The most important thing is to pay attention to the quality of the food you are eating rather than the quantity. If you focus on eating a healthy, balanced diet during your pregnancy rather than anxiously counting calories or, alternatively, embarking on a culinary free-for-all, then your weight gain should remain within the healthy range.

Recommended weight gain

Here is a rough guide to your recommended weight gain during pregnancy, taking into account your starting weight (see the BMI chart overleaf).

- For a woman in the healthy/normal range (BMI 20 25): a weight gain of 11–16 kg (25–35 lb).

- If you are overweight (BMI 25+): a weight gain of around 7 kg (15 lb).

- If you are underweight (BMI 19 and below): a weight gain up to 18 kg (40 lb).

Body Mass Index (BMI) chart

Weight	Height									
	1.47m (58 in)	1.52 m (60 in)	1.57 m (62 in)	1.62 m (64 in)	1.68 m (66 in)	1.73 m (68 in)	1.78 m (70 in)	1.83 m (72 in)	1.88 m (74 in)	1.93 m (76 in)
54 kg (120 lb)	25	24	22	21	19	18	17	16	15	15
57 kg (125 lb)	26	24	23	22	20	19	18	17	16	15
59 kg (130 lb)	27	25	24	22	21	20	19	18	17	16
61 kg (135 lb)	28	26	25	23	22	21	19	18	17	16
63 kg (140 lb)	29	27	26	24	23	21	20	19	18	17
66 kg (145 lb)	30	28	27	25	23	22	21	20	19	18
68 kg (150 lb)	31	29	28	26	24	23	22	20	19	18
70 kg (155 lb)	32	30	28	27	25	24	22	21	20	19
73 kg (160 lb)	34	31	29	28	26	24	23	22	21	20
75 kg (165 lb)	35	32	30	28	27	25	24	22	21	20
77 kg (170 lb)	36	33	31	29	28	26	24	23	22	21
79 kg (175 lb)	37	34	32	30	28	27	25	24	23	21
82 kg (180 lb)	38	35	33	31	29	27	26	24	23	22
84 kg (185 lb)	39	36	34	32	30	28	27	25	24	23
86 kg (190 lb)	40	37	35	33	31	29	27	26	24	23
88 kg (195 lb)	41	38	36	34	32	30	28	27	25	24
91 kg (200 lb)	42	39	37	34	32	30	29	27	26	24
93 kg (205 lb)	43	40	38	35	33	31	29	28	26	25
95 kg (210 lb)	44	41	39	36	34	32	30	29	27	26
98 kg (215 lb)	45	42	39	37	35	33	31	29	27	26
100 kg (220 lb)	46	43	40	38	36	34	32	30	28	27
102 kg (225 lb)	47	44	41	39	36	34	32	31	28	27
104 kg (230 lb)	48	45	42	40	37	35	33	31	29	28
107 kg (235 lb)	49	46	43	40	38	36	34	32	30	29
109 kg (240 lb)	50	47	44	41	39	36	35	33	31	29
111 kg (245 lb)	51	48	45	42	40	37	35	33	32	30

Please be aware that these are guidelines to help you achieve the optimum weight gain for you and your baby during pregnancy. Taking a balanced and flexible approach is more important than sticking rigorously to calorie guidelines. Both you and your baby will benefit from trying to remain within the upper and lower limits of the recommended weight gain.

Problems associated with excessive weight gain

As well as making your pregnancy more uncomfortable and having more weight to lose after the birth, there are other problems associated with excessive weight gain in pregnancy.

- Increased risk of high blood pressure.

- Increased risk of gestational diabetes.

- Increased risk of pre-eclampsia.

- Increased pressure on your back.

- Worsening varicose veins.

Problems associated with being underweight during pregnancy

Equally there are problems associated with gaining too little weight or being underweight during pregnancy.

- It can lead to low birth weight for your baby and the problems associated with that.

- It can lead to premature birth.

- There can be a lack of fat stores to enable breast-feeding after the birth.

● If your lack of weight gain is due to a poor diet or not eating enough, you and your baby will be missing out on vital nutrients.

Weight gain in pregnancy should be looked at on an individual basis, so if you are concerned it's a good idea to discuss it with your GP or midwife to get an accurate picture of what is healthy for you. You will also find useful calculators online that will give you a rough estimate.

What weight gain you can expect

It is important to remember that putting on weight in pregnancy isn't like putting on weight normally. Only around one-third of what you gain will be fat (3–4 kg/8–10 lb) and fat is there for a purpose: to provide energy stores for breast-feeding. One of the many advantages of breast-feeding for you is that it helps you regain your original shape and weight after your baby's birth – it contracts the uterus and uses up these fat stores. And the rest of the weight? Approximately a second third of the weight (4–5.5 kg/10–12 lb) will be made up of your baby, placenta and the amniotic fluid (giving birth is probably one of the only times you can lose almost a stone in weight overnight!).

The remaining third of the weight consists of:

● Extra body fluid: 1–1.5 kg (2.5–3 lb).

● Increased blood volume: 1–1.5 kg (2.5–3 lb).

● Increased breast weight: 450 g (1 lb).

● Expansion of your uterus: 1 kg (2.5 lb).

When can you expect to gain weight?

- In the first trimester you will only put on about 1–2 kg (2.5–4 lb).

- In the second trimester you can expect a weight gain of around 250–500 g (0.5–1 lb) per week.

- In the third trimester you can expect to gain weight at around the same rate. This is when you need those extra calories because this is when your baby is doing most of his growing. Between week 28 and week 40 he will grow an incredible 350 per cent, laying down his own fat stores, so that he is born at a healthy weight.

Good nutrition for you and your baby

During pregnancy your body has to cope with a great deal. Not only is it producing a brand-new human being, it is also changing and adapting to cope with the birth process and what will be required of it afterwards.

Women have evolved to have babies and down the centuries have simply relied on common sense and the handed-down advice of their mother and extended family for knowledge and information. However, now that we know so much more about what happens during pregnancy we have the ability to give our bodies a helping hand. We can supply the body with all the nutrients and fuel it needs to support us and our baby as well as possible.

Nutritional basics

At the very simplest level, you should aim to eat a diet that includes as wide a variety of fresh fruits and vegetables as possible to ensure you get as complete a range of vitamins, minerals and nutrients as you can.

Things you can do to stay healthy

- Make sure you stay fully hydrated: drinking about six to eight glasses of water a day should be enough.

- Never skip meals and try to keep healthy snacks on hand to maintain your energy levels and ward off fatigue and the nausea that often accompanies the early stages of pregnancy.

- Try not to rely on processed food and ready-meals and opt for home cooking as much as you can.

- Don't give yourself unrealistic expectations – no one can eat a perfect diet all the time.

Your pregnancy diet

Your pregnancy diet should be made up of approximately:

- 50–60 per cent carbohydrates.

- 25–35 per cent healthy fats.

- 20 per cent protein.

Carbohydrates

Carbohydrates are important in pregnancy as they provide the basic fuel for you and your baby: the energy he needs to grow. Carbohydrates break down into glucose in your bloodstream that crosses into the placenta. Your baby needs a nice, steady stream of glucose and you can provide this by eating complex and unrefined carbohydrates, which break down slowly – rather than refined starches or foods that contain a lot of sugar. These can lead to spikes and troughs in your blood-sugar levels and the amount of glucose your baby is receiving.

Try to limit your intake of white bread, pasta, rice, pastries and processed foods and replace them with wholegrain bread, brown rice, whole-wheat pasta, wholegrain cereals, oatmeal and sweet potatoes.

Fruits and vegetables are also excellent sources of carbohydrate, providing you with the fibre and vitamins you need. Try to make these, plus complex carbohydrates, the backbone of all your meals.

Protein

Protein is very important during pregnancy. It not only provides the building blocks for your baby, but it is vital for your health too. You need protein to help with the expansion of your uterus (which will grow to the size of a watermelon), for your increased blood volume and to help your breast development.

During pregnancy you need roughly 15 per cent more protein than the average daily requirement and this is easily achieved. Just by making sure you include some protein at every meal you will be getting an adequate supply.

Good sources of protein include: red meat, poultry, fish, cheese, tofu, eggs, nuts, beans and seeds.

Fats

Not all fat is bad for you. In fact fats play an important role in your baby's development and the overall maintenance of your own health. As a general guideline, between 25 and 35 per cent of the daily calories you consume should be derived from healthy fats. See page 48 for a closer look at which fats are most beneficial and why.

Vitamin supplements

Although you should be able to get all the vitamins and minerals you and your baby need from your normal, everyday food, there is no harm in making quite certain that your body has what it needs – just to be sure. Eat a well-rounded diet and take an approved pregnancy supplement (your chemist or midwife should be able to advise you). Your diet should include folic acid and vitamin D, but NOT vitamin A, which can be harmful if it is taken in too large quantities during pregnancy (see page 52). Women of South Asian, African or Middle Eastern origin, or those who have limited exposure to the sun, should also take a vitamin D supplement. These are available from your midwife. Talk to your GP or midwife if you need more advice about which supplements are best suited to your needs.

Vitamins and minerals

Along with the basic requirements of a healthy diet there are a few special considerations to be aware of when you are pregnant. Here is a list of the vitamins and minerals that you need more of during your pregnancy: some are for your benefit and some are for the benefit of your growing baby.

Although amounts and percentages are mentioned, try not to worry too much about these. It's more important to incorporate these foods into your daily diet, rather than slavishly measuring out and worrying about serving sizes. Combine this information with the rough guidelines for your intake of carbohydrates, proteins and fat and a pregnancy supplement on the previous pages, and you can be confident that you and your baby are getting exactly what you both need.

Folic acid

When: When trying to conceive; the first trimester.

Why: Folic acid is known to significantly reduce the risk of neural tube defects, such as spina bifida, by up to 70 per cent.

In the first few weeks of your pregnancy your baby's nervous system is developing, which in turn goes on to help the development of his other systems. This is why it's so important to ensure you take enough folic acid early on in pregnancy for at least the first 12 weeks.

How: Take an additional folic acid supplement of at least 400 mg a day to ensure you are getting enough of this crucial vitamin; if you can start taking it before you conceive, so much the better.

Try to eat food that is rich in folates, such as beans and legumes, dark leafy vegetables, fortified cereals, citrus fruit, broccoli, avocado, beetroot and asparagus.

Vitamin D

When: Throughout pregnancy and breastfeeding.

Why: Your baby needs vitamin D to develop healthy teeth and bones. Vitamin D supplements are recommended because many women have low levels due to a lack of exposure to the sun or a diet that is low in vitamin D. Women particularly at risk of vitamin D deficiency include:

- Women of South Asian, African, Caribbean or Middle Eastern origin.
- Women with limited exposure to sunlight.
- Women who have a diet low in vitamin D (who consume no oily fish, eggs, meat or fortified cereal).
- Women with a BMI of over 30.

How: Healthy Start vitamin supplements are available, which provide the 10 micrograms of vitamin D you need per day. Vitamin D can be found naturally in oily fish, eggs, meat and fortified cereals.

Iron

When: Throughout pregnancy, particularly during the third trimester.

Why: Your body needs iron to produce haemoglobin, the chemical that carries oxygen in your blood. When you are pregnant your blood volume increases significantly (you will have almost 50 per cent more by the end of your pregnancy) and therefore you need more iron. Your baby will make sure his iron needs are met, so if you don't consume enough for both of you, you will be left feeling tired and weak, perhaps even anaemic. If you are found to be deficient you will need to consume substances high in iron.

How: Your body is most efficient at absorbing the iron it needs from animal products, especially red meat, sardines and poultry (dark meat). If you don't eat those foods you can find iron in pulses, dried fruit and dark, leafy vegetables.

Calcium

When: Towards the end of the second trimester and throughout the third trimester.

Why: Calcium is used in the formation of bone. From around week 26 your baby will need more calcium because his skeleton, bones and teeth are being formed. Calcium is also important for blood clotting, developing your baby's heartbeat, muscle and nerve function.

As with iron, your baby will be sure to take all the calcium he needs, and it's important that you have enough in your system so that you are not deprived. If you don't have enough calcium in your blood, your body will start taking it from your bone reserves, and this can lead to problems for you later on as well as increasing your risk of osteoporosis.

How: Your recommended calcium intake is 800 mg a day. Try to get this from low-fat dairy products such as yogurt, cheese and milk. It is also important that you get enough vitamin D to aid the absorption of calcium.

Other sources of calcium include green, leafy vegetables, tofu, broccoli, tinned salmon and calcium-fortified orange juice.

Heart-healthy fats

When: Throughout pregnancy, especially during the second and third trimesters.

Why: There is growing evidence that what you eat during pregnancy can set your baby up to have a healthy cardiovascular system in the future. In the same way that certain fats are bad for the heart, consuming high amounts of these could increase your baby's risk of developing problems later on in life.

How: Choose unsaturated and monosaturated fats such as olive oil and sunflower oil. Avoid margarine, processed foods and don't overdo full-fat dairy products or beef.

Hints for a healthy, balanced diet

During pregnancy you should eat a healthy, balanced diet similar to the optimum diet for general health.

- Aim to divide your meals as follows: 50–60 per cent carbohydrates, 25–35 per cent healthy fats, 20 per cent protein.

- Look at the above lists of foods that are particularly important during pregnancy (see pages 42–8) and try to incorporate as many of those into your diet as possible.

- Eat as many freshly prepared meals as possible and avoid highly processed and 'junk' food as much as you can.

- Concentrate on eating a wide range of foods and include as many fresh vegetables and fruits as possible.

- Keep your fluid intake up – plain, fresh water is the best choice (limit caffeine-containing drinks such as tea, coffee and fizzy drinks and avoid alcoholic drinks).

- Avoid certain foods and take care with others (see below).

- Take a well-rounded pregnancy vitamin supplement throughout your pregnancy (and a separate folic acid supplement in the first trimester).

Foods and drinks to avoid and limit

We all occasionally indulge in things we know aren't strictly good for us: one too many glasses of wine, a junk-food takeaway with all the extras or a slice of chocolate cake, and there's really no need to feel guilty about the odd indulgence. However, during pregnancy it's important to take more care than usual about what you eat and drink.

Here is a list of foods that you should limit or avoid during pregnancy. With some items it is a matter of personal choice, but others should be strictly avoided during pregnancy. These are foods that can damage your unborn baby if you eat them just once – not because they are intrinsically bad, but because they are a common source of food poisoning.

Foods to avoid completely

- Unpasteurised cheeses.

- Mould-ripened cheeses such as Brie and Camembert.

- Soft blue-veined cheeses.

- Pâté – including vegetable pâté.

- Raw eggs or anything made with raw or partially cooked eggs.

- Unpasteurised milk, including goat and sheep's milk.

- Raw meat or poultry.

- Raw seafood – including shellfish. (Sushi that includes previously frozen fish should be safe – if you are unsure of its origins it's best to err on the side of caution and avoid eating it.)

- Pre-prepared salads.

- Unwashed fruit or vegetables.

All the foods in the list (see above) have higher incidences of listeria, which is a bacteria that can cause food poisoning – and pregnant women are 20 times more likely to contract listeriosis because of their lowered immune systems. Although it is rare, the incidence rate among pregnant women is 12 in 100,000, compared to 0.7 in 100,000 among the general population. Real caution must be taken because the effects can be devastating (it can infect the placenta, the amniotic fluid and the baby, even causing miscarriage or stillbirth and newborn babies can be born with listeria infections, which can lead to death).

The best advice is to avoid these foods in pregnancy because the risks simply aren't worth taking. However, if you eat any of them without being aware of it, for example when you are in a restaurant, don't panic. The likelihood of a mouthful of one of these foods developing into listeriosis is really very rare. However, if you find yourself experiencing flu-like symptoms or a mild temperature, then do contact your GP simply as a precaution and, if you feel fine, just get on with your day without worrying or feeling guilty.

In some countries women are advised not to eat cold meats or smoked fish to avoid listeria poisoning. These are considered safe in the UK, but avoid them if you are concerned and take extra care when you are abroad.

Alcohol

There is continuing controversy over alcohol and pregnancy and the current government and NHS guidelines are that you should avoid drinking alcohol in the first three months, in particular, to reduce the risk of miscarriage and then, if possible, during the rest of your pregnancy too.

If you do choose to have the occasional drink, it's important to keep drinking under control. You should have no more than one to two units of alcohol (half a pint of beer or a very small glass of wine), and no more than once or twice a week. This is because excessive drinking in pregnancy can affect your baby's development, leading to low birth weight and heart defects as well as behavioural and learning disorders. At the more extreme end of the spectrum alcohol can cause foetal alcohol syndrome, which is the biggest cause of non-genetic mental handicap in the Western world.

Having a social life

If you are used to going out for drinks with friends or for work events, you will still want to join in socially during your pregnancy. You can easily substitute non-alcoholic drinks, such as fruit juices, for your usual tipple. If you do not want people to guess why you are not drinking early in your pregnancy or start asking questions, you could always say that you are on a health kick, or you could just pick a drink that looks just like an alcoholic drink – no one will be any the wiser.

Caffeine

Consuming high levels of caffeine in pregnancy can lead to a low birth weight, which is associated with further health problems for your baby. In extreme cases excessive caffeine consumption has also been linked to miscarriage.

The recommendation is that when you are pregnant you should not consume more than 200–300 mg of caffeine a day. That's roughly the equivalent of two cups of filter coffee or two or three cups of tea.

Don't forget that caffeine is also present in many soft drinks, particularly 'energy' drinks, and that it pops up in items such as chocolate and some cold and flu medications.

If you are a really dedicated coffee-drinker, you will need to investigate alternatives. You can try decaffeinated coffees and teas, but do bear in mind that almost all of these contain small amounts of caffeine. Why not try herbal, green and black teas? Also some people swear by sipping cups of hot water – it may sound dull, but you do get used to it and it can make a comforting hot drink.

Foods containing vitamin A

We all think of vitamins being intrinsically 'good' for us, but during pregnancy, especially in early pregnancy, high levels of vitamin A can cause birth defects and liver toxicity. To lower the risk of this:

● Avoid liver and liver products such as pâté or liver-based sausages.

● Be careful not to take vitamin supplements (including some fish oil supplements) that contain high levels of vitamin A.

Fish to avoid

The reason pregnant women are encouraged to limit their intake of certain types of fish is because of a possible build-up of mercury in them, which can have a negative effect on the baby's developing nervous system. Fish known to have higher levels of mercury and therefore best eaten sparingly during pregnancy are:

- Swordfish.

- Marlin.

- Shark.

Try to limit your intake of the following oily fish to two portions or less a week:

- Tuna (up to four medium cans of tuna is fine).

- Mackerel.

- Sardines.

- Trout.

Saturated and trans-fats

These types of fats aren't great at the best of times because of the effects they can have on the heart. Evidence suggests that you can lower your baby's risk of cardiovascular disease later in life by cutting back on them during pregnancy. Try to limit your intake of:

- Beef.

- Full-fat dairy (though be sure to keep up your calcium intake).

- Margarine.

- Baked goods.

- Ready-meals containing high levels of preservatives, artificial flavourings and colourings, added salt and sugar and 'junk' food such as commercially made burgers, fries and battered chicken.

Extra care with hygiene

During pregnancy it is worth taking a little extra care when it comes to the common-sense hygiene rules in the kitchen. When you are pregnant your immune system changes because its first priority is your baby, making you more susceptible to infection. So be sure to:

- Wash your hands before preparing food.

- Wash all fruits and vegetables.

- Keep work surfaces disinfected.

- Use separate chopping boards, knives and preparation areas for meat, to avoid potential cross-contamination.

- Store all food correctly. For example, always cover foods you place in the fridge with cling film and always place uncooked meats on shelves below other foods, to avoid the possibility of contamination via dripping liquids.

- Try to be vigilant and check all sell-by and best-before dates on food packaging. Don't eat food that has gone past its dates.

- Make sure that all ready-meals and reheated foods are thoroughly cooked through. They must be piping hot before you eat them.

Toxoplasmosis

The parasite toxoplasmosis can also have a devastating effect in pregnancy, especially if you contract it during the first trimester. (See page 188 for more on this.) To limit the risk of infection be sure to:

- Cook all beef, pork and lamb to at least medium, preferably well done. And avoid eating rare or 'blue' meat altogether.

- Wash all fruit, vegetables and salads thoroughly to remove any traces of soil, which can carry toxoplasma.

Salmonella

Salmonella can cause vomiting, high fever, diarrhoea and dehydration in the mother, though it does not directly harm the baby. However, it is still not pleasant and is best avoided by:

- Avoiding raw eggs or products that might contain them such as homemade mayonnaise.

- Making sure that all chicken is completely cooked through.

Eating a healthy diet and avoiding foods high in fat and salt is an easy way to provide your unborn baby with the best start in life. It has the added bonus of being good for you too! Eating well is a way of caring for yourself and your baby during your pregnancy. You may want to continue your healthy diet after your baby has arrived.

4
Caring for Yourself During Pregnancy

A healthy diet, as seen in the previous chapter, is vital for maintaining a healthy pregnancy, but you will also need to look after your body in other ways. During pregnancy, the many changes it goes through will put your body under a certain amount of strain, and it's a good idea to try to ensure that you don't experience any unnecessary difficulties.

You will also want to think more carefully about things you do that may affect your body and your baby while you are pregnant. You may find that you have questions or concerns about whether certain things are safe or recommended during pregnancy, and many of these issues will be addressed in this chapter. If you are unsure about anything, ask your GP or midwife.

Caring for your teeth

During pregnancy you are more susceptible to suffering from gum disease because of increased blood flow and hormone levels in your body. Almost half of all pregnant women in the UK can expect to experience some form of gingivitis. You'll know that this is happening to you if you start noticing that your gums are swollen or that they bleed when you brush and floss.

Chronic gum disease in pregnancy has been linked to premature birth and low birth weight, so it pays to take a bit more care and attention when it comes to your oral health during the nine months of pregnancy.

Dental health issues

When you're pregnant, your teeth need special care. In addition to your usual dental hygiene routine, here are some things you should think about.

- Dental care is free when you are pregnant and for the first year after your baby's birth, so be sure to attend regular appointments so that you can keep an eye on everything.

- Regular cleaning by your dentist or hygienist will help to prevent gum problems developing. Be sure to tell them that you are pregnant so that they can modify any treatment accordingly.

- Your dentist probably won't recommend mercury fillings, but to be on the safe side ask for alternatives to fillings that might contain mercury, as they are not safe.

- Maintain high standards of oral hygiene at home every day: floss and brush thoroughly at least twice a day.

- If you are suffering from pregnancy sickness (vomiting) resist the temptation to brush your teeth immediately afterwards. The stomach acid makes your teeth more vulnerable than normal. It is better to rinse your mouth with water or an appropriate mouth-wash instead.

● Be sure to eat a healthy diet that provides you with enough calcium and vitamin D to keep your teeth strong and help your growing baby develop strong teeth and bones.

Foot care during pregnancy

Pregnancy puts a lot of pressure on your joints so it is very important to wear supportive footwear to avoid foot, leg and back problems. High heels are unsuitable as they put unnecessary pressure on your back and knees when they are already under strain. Entirely flat shoes, such as flip-flops or ballet flats, are also unsuitable as they don't give your feet the necessary support. You should choose well-fitting, supportive shoes, ideally with a strap or laces.

The Society of Chiropodists and Podiatrists gives the following advice for healthy feet in pregnancy:

● Choose supportive footwear with a supportive arch, a firm heel and extra shock absorption.

● Choose a heel height of 3 cm (1.2 in), as this shifts the weight further forward onto your feet, which can help alleviate any discomfort.

● Choose shoes with a rounded or square-shaped toe rather than a pointed one. The toe should be high enough and wide enough to comfortably fit your toes. Make sure there is 1 cm between the longest toe and the end of the shoe.

- Pick a shoe with a strap to keep it firmly on your foot. It's best to avoid fiddly straps that are difficult to do up – especially in your final trimester.

- Feet swell during the day, so it's best to buy shoes later in the day when your feet are at their largest.

- Keep active. Keep your lower limbs moving, even while you are resting. Avoid crossing your legs or ankles when sitting.

If you are suffering from swelling of the ankles and feet, try resting for an hour a day with your feet elevated. You can also do foot exercises to help reduce the swelling – try bending and stretching your foot up and down 30 times, then rotating your feet in a circle eight times one way, then eight times the other way. (See page 154 for more on this.)

Wearing a seat belt

As your bump grows you may find seat belts start to get a bit uncomfortable, but it's crucial that you fasten the belt securely and tightly to protect both you and your baby. You should position the lap portion of the belt as low as possible so it sits under your bump and across your thighs and hips. (Never position the belt across or above your belly, as this could hurt your baby). The shoulder portion should be positioned between your breasts with the side of the strap around the side of your bump. For more information on wearing a seat belt and safety during pregnancy, see: http://think.direct.gov.uk.

Looking after your hair

You may notice that your hair has become fuller and thicker during your pregnancy. This can be a blessing or a curse, depending on what your hair was like originally. It's all down to hormones.

Hormones and your hair

High levels of pregnancy hormones mean that the growth phase of your normal hair cycle is increased and your hair will become thicker, grow faster and be more lustrous. After the birth these levels return to normal and the effects are reversed. You may feel that you are losing more hair than normal at this point, but this is probably in contrast with the last few months of pregnancy. Most women find that they start to lose their hair around four to five months after the delivery. Hormones can affect the hair in other ways too. You may experience a change in texture: it may change from fine to coarse, from straight to curly and vice versa. Use products that are intended for your 'new' hair type and, if you don't like it, comfort yourself with the fact that it will soon be back to normal after the birth.

Hair colourants and perms

Women used to be told not to dye or perm their hair during pregnancy. This was because of concerns about the chemicals in certain dyes and perming fluids. Evidence suggests that it is probably fine to dye and perm your hair due to the low levels of chemicals you actually come into contact with.

If you are concerned:

- Hold off dyeing your hair until after the first trimester.

- Use dyes that don't come into direct contact with your scalp, so perhaps opt for highlights rather than having an all-over colour.

- If you are dyeing your hair at home, be sure to do so in a well-ventilated area and wear rubber gloves.

- Consider using vegetable-based, semi-permanent dyes such as henna instead of chemical ones.

Be aware that due to the difference in your hair's texture during pregnancy, you might have a very different look to your normal one. For this reason, some hairdressers choose not to perform perms on pregnant women, not because they are worried about safety, but because they can't predict the end result.

A last word should go to the Brazilian blow-dry or keratin treatment. These have become very popular in recent years and there are several different varieties, using different chemical formulations, available. Most manufacturers do not endorse their products as being suitable for use during pregnancy and breast-feeding, simply because they have not yet done the research to establish their safety.

Body hair

While you might appreciate the extra volume pregnancy is adding to the hair on your head, you probably won't be pleased that it's doing the same elsewhere to hair on your body. Some women do notice an increase in body and facial hair. As well as random hairs popping up in unexpected places, such as on your breasts or stomach, you may find that they are coarser and darker than normal.

Fortunately this hair growth is temporary and you should find that the problem subsides after your baby's birth. Be patient, though, as it can take up to six months for your hormones to settle back to their normal levels.

In the meantime, if excess hair is bothering you, the best advice is to tweeze stray hairs or wax larger areas. Always check the instructions on the packaging before you use depilatory creams or bleaches in case they are not recommended for use during pregnancy.

Looking after your skin

The 'glow' of pregnancy is well known and it's true that some women do seem to 'bloom' during this time. A combination of extra fluid, increased blood flow and extra oil production can leave the skin looking plumper, more supple, energised and 'dewy'.

However, not all the effects of pregnancy on the skin are so desirable. How your skin reacts depends on several different factors. There may be a genetic component, so if your own mother or sister were particularly susceptible to stretch marks, for example, prepare for the same to happen to you. Equally, if you've noticed that you tend to suffer from hormone-related breakouts of spots just before your period is due you may find that your skin reacts similarly in pregnancy, especially during the first trimester. Your skin may also be much more sensitive to sun and burning, which may produce uneven pigmentation.

Common skin changes during pregnancy

Stretch marks

Most women get stretch marks during pregnancy. Not only is your skin stretching further and faster than ever before but, thanks to pregnancy hormones, it contains less collagen, making it more fragile and susceptible to tearing.

Stretch marks appear as fine red, pink or purplish lines that spread across the abdomen, thighs, breasts, hips or anywhere there has been rapid growth. The good news is that, given time, they will fade considerably, eventually turning to a pale silvery colour and barely visible.

There's not much you can do to prevent stretch marks developing: how many you get and how severe they are depends on your skin and body type. All you can do is try to ensure a slow, steady, gradual weight gain during pregnancy. Many women swear by applying special oils or creams (specifically vitamin E creams) as a preventative measure. There isn't much evidence to suggest that this works, but it can't do any harm and keeping the skin moisturised is always a plus. (For more on this, see page 160.)

Changes in skin pigmentation

Pigmentation changes during pregnancy are brought about by your hormones. While you are pregnant you will notice that areas of skin pigmentation such as moles, freckles and birthmarks will appear darker. You might also develop a few extra moles and a darkening of the skin in other areas. Areas commonly affected include genitals, armpits, legs and hands. Dark areas should fade gradually after your baby is born.

Quite early on in your pregnancy, your nipples and areolae (the circular area around your nipples) will also darken. There is a theory that this helps the baby find the breast when he is feeding. Unlike other hormonal pigmentation changes most women find that, although they may fade somewhat, their nipples and areola remain darker than they were before pregnancy.

Linea nigra

At some point around the second trimester you may notice a dark vertical line appearing on your stomach. Known as the 'linea nigra', it runs the length of the stomach, bisecting it. This line is, in fact, always there, but it is normally so faint that we don't notice it. In pregnancy hormonal changes make it darker and more visible. Like most other pigmentation changes it will fade after pregnancy, but it might take a little longer to disappear completely. Exposure to the sun may make it look even darker.

The 'mask of pregnancy'

This change in facial pigmentation is known as the 'mask of pregnancy', but the medical term is 'chloasma'. Depending on your skin tone, you may develop darker or lighter patches of pigmentation around your forehead, nose and cheeks. The 'mask' is more common in women with darker skin tones. If you do develop it, be assured that it will fade after your baby is born. In the meantime your best option is to use extra foundation or concealer to try to give your skin an even appearance. You can buy concealer that is designed for hiding birthmarks and this might work better than your usual version. Stay out of the sun and always wear a high sun protection factor sun cream because exposure to the sun can exacerbate the condition. Make sure you are getting enough folic acid in your diet from green, leafy vegetables and your pregnancy supplement (see page 44) as hyper-pigmentation has been connected to folate deficiency.

Spots

If you had a tendency to get hormone-related breakouts of spots prior to becoming pregnant you may find that the same thing happens now. It is quite common to experience mild or moderate acne during pregnancy, especially during the first trimester. Try to look after your skin by using mild washes and scrubs that are suitable for sensitive skin and won't exacerbate or encourage excess oil production. An oil-free moisturiser is also a good idea. If you can, try to use organic products.

Be aware that some acne medications are not suitable to be used during pregnancy as they can cause complications with foetal development. Most oral medications are not advised during pregnancy and topical medications should also be avoided, especially those containing vitamin A and other retinoids. Do not use any of these before speaking to your GP, who will advise you on the best course of action for treating acne. And, remember, your skin will return to normal after your baby is born.

Skin tags

Skin tags are little protruding growths of skin. About the size of a grain of rice, they tend to form in areas where there is a lot of friction or additional moisture, so arm pits, the areas beneath your breasts, your groin area and sometimes around your neck are common places to find them. Skin tags become more common as we get older, but they are harmless and often not particularly disfiguring. Sometimes they fall off of their own accord after pregnancy. If they bother you, speak to a dermatologist about getting them removed.

Spider veins

You might find that 'spider veins', which are small thread-like veins that are red or bluish in colour, appear during pregnancy. Commonly found on the face and legs, they are caused by a combination of hormones, increased blood flow and circulatory changes.

These veins should go after the birth, but if they bother you there are ways you can have them removed (after your baby is born) that you can discuss with your GP.

During your pregnancy, gentle exercise, a high-fibre diet full of vitamin C, making sure you don't sit or stand for long stretches of time and using support stockings all go some way towards preventing the formation of spider veins.

Rashes

As well as heat rash, pregnant women can suffer from PUPP (pruritic urticarial papules and plaques of pregnancy), which is an itchy, raised, bumpy red rash, normally appearing during the third trimester. It is relatively rare, occurring in less than one per cent of pregnancies. As with other rashes, try your best not to scratch and treat it with soothing baths and cold compresses.

Red palms and soles

The majority of women experience a reddening of the palms of their hands and soles of their feet during pregnancy. This is caused by hormones and increased blood volume and is harmless, though it can be a little itchy and uncomfortable. Try cooling your hands to alleviate the irritation.

Skin care guidelines

- During pregnancy you should be able to follow your usual skin-care routine, making adjustments only if necessary.

- Try to avoid using soaps or face washes that contain astringents, as these can increase oil production, which is already working overtime during your pregnancy. For the same reason, opt for an oil-free, non-comedogenic moisturiser.

- If you can find, and afford, products with natural or organic ingredients, choose these. That way you can limit the amount of chemicals being absorbed through the skin.

- Check what your usual moisturisers, face washes and scrubs contain. Avoid using products that contain BHA, salicylic acids or vitamin A.

- Avoid taking hot baths. They are not beneficial for your skin and can exacerbate some of the problems associated with skin during pregnancy. (You should also avoid using saunas, Jacuzzis and steam rooms during pregnancy because of the risks of overheating, dehydration and fainting.)

- Consider avoiding the sun, or wear sun protection or a hat.

Sun protection during pregnancy

Much as we love the sun, pregnancy is not the right time for sun-worshipping. Your skin is more sensitive than usual and it can be more prone to burning and pigmentation changes, which might not always be temporary. However, you don't need to stay out of the sun completely as vitamin D is good for you, but be sure to take sensible precautions. There have been recent reports about pregnant women avoiding certain sun-protection creams because they contain vitamin A (as high levels can be harmful to pregnant women – see page 52). However the consensus is that the benefits of sun protection far outweigh any possible risks from chemicals that might be absorbed through your skin.

Due to your increased body size, greater blood flow and pregnancy hormones, it is easy to overheat in hot climates and become dehydrated when you are pregnant. Neither of these is good for you or your baby. While the vitamin D you get from the sun helps your absorption of calcium, sun exposure can lower your levels of folic acid, which is important during pregnancy (see page 18 for more on this).

Tips for being exposed to the sun

- Always wear a good-quality UVA/UVB sunscreen of factor 30 or above – your skin may be extra sensitive to the sun during pregnancy.

- Try to keep your face shaded with a broad-brimmed hat and cover up other parts of your body too, especially if you have chloasma (see page 65). The sun will make any dark patches on your skin appear even darker.

- Keep out of the sun at the hottest time of the day, which is normally between 11am and 2pm, but in hotter countries this period of time can be far longer.

- Avoid overheating and dehydration. Be sure to drink enough water and take frequent dips in the pool (if you are on holiday) to cool off or have a cool shower or bath. If you feel hot or unwell, get into the shade as soon as possible.

- If you are in the later stages of pregnancy do not lie on your back to sunbathe (see page 74).

- Never use sun beds when you are pregnant. Your skin may be more sensitive during this time and it is more likely to burn. Some sun beds emit larger doses of UV rays than ordinary Mediterranean-strength sunlight and studies have found that there is a possible link between UV rays and folic acid deficiency because UV rays can break down folic acid.

Botox

Botox is popular, but using it when you are pregnant is not recommended, especially if it is purely for cosmetic purposes. There haven't yet been enough studies done into its possible effects to be able to make a judgement on its safety or otherwise, so it is best not to use it.

If you had Botox treatment before you realised you were pregnant don't worry, as it is highly unlikely that such small amounts injected directly into the muscle will have caused any problems. If you need Botox for medical reasons talk to your GP and weigh up the advantages and disadvantages. If you are considering Botox for purely cosmetic reasons, it's best to hold off until after you've had your baby and have finished breast-feeding.

It's interesting to know that one of the plus aspects of pregnancy is that it is 'nature's Botox': all the extra fluid coursing around your body leaves your skin plumper and firmer, fine lines and wrinkles appear diminished and the increased blood flow gives you that pregnancy 'glow' (see page 63).

Tattoos

Getting a tattoo when you are pregnant is unlikely to cause you or your baby any serious problems, but it's sensible not to take any risks. After all, the tattoo is going to be with you for life, so it's probably better to wait until after your baby is born. Not only will it be a lot more comfortable when you have it done, but also the risk of contracting hepatitis B or HIV will be limited to just you, your immune system will be better equipped to fight off any resulting minor infections and you won't have to worry about the (very small) chance that the chemical dyes could affect your unborn baby.

Most tattooists won't tattoo pregnant women. However, if you really are determined to get a tattoo while you are pregnant, make sure that you find a licensed tattoo artist who is happy to do the work and be certain to inform them that you're pregnant, even if you aren't showing yet. Check that the tattooist is wearing gloves and using sterile equipment and fresh disposable needles from an unopened packet.

Body piercing

It's best to wait until after your pregnancy before getting any new piercings. When you are pregnant your immune system is lowered, leaving you less able to fight off any resulting infections. It will also take your body longer to heal. Most respectable body piercers will tell you to come back a couple of months after you've had your baby and after you have finished breast-feeding.

If you already have body piercings, these can be affected by your pregnancy.

Existing piercings

While there are no medical reasons to take out your piercings during pregnancy, you may find they become uncomfortable, especially nipple or clitoral piercings as these areas are likely to become more sensitive. Talk to your piercer about flexible rings or special bars to keep your piercing open.

- Belly button: as your bump gets bigger you might find it difficult to keep the piercing in. If a Caesarean section is necessary, you will be asked to remove your piercing or tape it down.

- Clitoris: piercings need to be removed before giving birth.

- Nipple: piercings will have to be removed before breast-feeding.

Sleep

You may be prepared for the lack of sleep that comes with having a newborn baby, but you may not have factored in how sleep-deprived you might be before you get to that stage.

Pregnancy, especially in the later stages, can throw up sleep issues of its own. Just because you know it's time for bed, it doesn't mean that your unborn baby does and his movements and metabolism might not necessarily correspond with yours. Combine this with problems getting comfortable, needing to go to the bathroom frequently, restless legs (see page 75), heartburn (see page 77) and any general anxiety and it can be hard to drop off at night.

Try to get in as much sleep as you can before the birth. You probably need at least eight hours a night as well as naps during the day, if possible. If you can't fit in a nap, trying lying down for five minutes with your feet elevated slightly – you'll find it will do wonders.

Help yourself sleep at night

Here are some general guidelines if you are suffering from pregnancy-related insomnia:

Pregnancy-related insomnia

● Try to stick to the same routine every bedtime. It will calm your mind and your body can prepare for sleep.

● Have a warm bath and put a few drops of relaxing oils, such as lavender, into it.

● Don't have any caffeine after midday. This includes all caffeine-containing food and drink items such as chocolate and fizzy drinks as well as coffee.

- Have a warm, milky drink or soothing herbal tea to help you feel sleepy before you go to bed.

- Take gentle exercise earlier on in the day – not just before bed as this can stimulate you rather than calm you down.

- Switch off the TV and computer an hour before you are planning to go to sleep, otherwise your brain may remain overstimulated.

Find a comfortable position

You will probably find that, from quite early on in your pregnancy, sleeping on your front becomes uncomfortable. This is not just because of your growing bump, but because of breast tenderness and swelling.

Once you reach your second trimester, doctors recommend that you no longer sleep on your back. This is because the weight of your baby can put pressure on your vena cava vein, the main vein transporting blood to the heart. This can lead to a drop in blood pressure and a reduction in blood flow to the placenta. The best position to lie in is on your left-hand side as this optimises the blood flow to the placenta.

This side is preferable to the right as it allows the blood to flow freely to the kidneys and placenta and it ensures that your liver isn't being pressed on by your uterus. It's a good idea to try to get used to this position early on in pregnancy as it will make it easier to adapt to it later.

Use pillows

Pillows are your friend! Try putting one or two between your knees when you sleep or rest your bent leg on top of them. You can buy pregnancy 'wedges', which are soft, foam, wedge-shaped cushions designed to go under your bump to alleviate the pressure. You can also get long-shaped pillows that run the length of your body. You put them between your legs, then under your bump and rest your head on the top end. You can also use this style of pillow to wrap around you when you are breast-feeding in bed after the birth.

Night-time annoyances

As well as finding it difficult to get to sleep, there may be other things that affect your sleep during the night. Some of these – such as needing to go to the bathroom more frequently – can be experienced during the daytime too, but of course they are much more annoying if they wake you up during the night!

Needing to go to the bathroom

You'll find frequent trips to the bathroom during the night become part of your life, especially during the first and third trimesters, when first your uterus and then your baby will be pressing down on your bladder. There's nothing much you can do about this apart from trying to cut back on fluids in the run-up to bedtime. However, be sure to compensate by drinking more fluids earlier in the day, as it is important to avoid becoming dehydrated.

Restless legs

Restless legs syndrome is that irritating need to move or flex your legs, which sometimes occurs when you are trying to drop off to sleep. It is relatively common during pregnancy, with up to one-quarter of all women experiencing it. Symptoms tend to be at their worst from the end of the third trimester onwards, but they should taper off after your baby is born. Try lessening its effects by exercising and stretching regularly throughout the day to improve your circulation. Also cut down on your caffeine intake and consider taking iron supplements, as restless legs syndrome has been linked to anaemia (see page 178).

Leg cramps

Anyone who has woken up from sleep clutching their calf knows the agony of night-time leg cramps.

Cramps may start to affect you towards the end of the second trimester. They are thought to be caused by a combination of the extra weight you are carrying and circulation issues. Calcium and magnesium deficiencies have also been blamed, but there is no real evidence for this.

To help prevent cramps at night be sure to:

- Keep your circulation going with regular, gentle exercise (see Chapter 5). Even taking a daily walk around the block can help.

- Stretch your calves throughout the day, flexing and rotating your ankles.

- Avoid sitting or standing for prolonged periods.

- Take a warm bath before bed to relax the muscles.

- Make sure you are drinking plenty of fluids during the day.

> **Warning**
>
> If your cramp is in one leg only and is persistent and if the leg is swollen, it is important you see your GP to make sure that you do not have a deep-vein thrombosis.

Heartburn

Heartburn is common in pregnancy and is caused by the effects of the hormone progesterone on your body and your baby growing and pushing against your stomach. It can be particularly troublesome at night when you are trying to get to sleep.

Keep night-time heartburn at bay

- Limit food and drinks that may aggravate it: alcohol (which should be avoided anyway), fizzy drinks, spicy foods, chocolate, citrus fruit and juices, rich or fatty foods, which are hard on your digestion.

- Avoid acidic foods such as vinegar.

- Try to eat small meals at regular intervals throughout the day rather than widely spaced heavy meals, especially before bedtime.

- Some pregnant women find that a milky drink helps, while others find that slightly flat sparkling water is good. Or you could try herbal tea.

- It may help indigestion to sleep with your upper body slightly raised, and you can do this with the help of pillows.

Nausea

Nausea is very common and one of the early signs of pregnancy (see page 144). It can be quite debilitating and come on all of a sudden, and for many women it is not confined to morning. If nausea is keeping you awake at night:

- Try keeping dry biscuits by your bed to nibble on if nausea strikes – especially when you first wake up in the morning.

- Ginger tea is thought to help.

Dreams

It is very common to experience particularly vivid dreams during pregnancy, which may wake you at night. You may find that this escalates as the birth approaches. This phenomenon is thought to be caused by a combination of progesterone, understandable anxiety, heightened emotions and the fact that because our sleep is disturbed during pregnancy we find ourselves in the dream portion of the sleep cycle more often (or we are more likely to remember our dreams as we keep waking up during them).

Worry

It is only natural that with the impending birth of a new baby you'll have a lot on your mind. You may be so busy that you do not get the chance to think about the life-changing event of your pregnancy until you go to bed, which is when worrying may well hit you. If you find it hard to wind down and let go at bedtime, follow these general guidelines for insomnia during pregnancy.

- You may find it helpful to try relaxation and breathing exercises (see opposite).

● Pregnancy yoga can be useful for centring yourself and calming the mind (see page 97).

● Keep a notebook and pencil by your bed. When a thought or an urgent 'to do' pops into your mind you can write it down and deal with it in the morning. That way the effort of remembering it won't keep you awake.

● Sometimes when you can't sleep it is better not to keep on trying. Instead, switch the light on and try to distract yourself with a good book until you feel drowsy again. However, beware of reading anything that stimulates your brain too much.

Relaxation visualisation for pregnancy

Sit in a quiet place, relax and close your eyes. Imagine that you are in a relaxing, familiar place you love. Perhaps it is in nature (for example, on a beach or in a flower-filled meadow).

Focus on this chosen location, using as many of your senses as you can. Feel the sand under your feet, smell the flowers, see the glistening water. You will feel calm and relaxed – let this feeling wash through you.

Breathing exercise for pregnancy

Maximise the flow of oxygen to your baby with this easy breathing exercise. It will help to calm you down if you are feeling a little stressed.

● Sit comfortably in a quiet place, with your back straight and eyes closed.

- Breathe in through your nose for a count of five and let as much air as possible fill you – expanding your abdomen.

- Hold the breath briefly and then release it through your mouth.

- Repeat this breathing pattern until you feel calm and serene again.

Intimacy during pregnancy

During the course of a normal, low-risk pregnancy there is no medical reason why you should abstain from sex, though you may not necessarily feel in the mood for it. There is no need to worry that sex could harm your baby or that he somehow 'knows' what is going on: he doesn't! However, you need to be aware that sex, and particularly orgasms, can cause some minor uterine contractions and even Braxton Hicks contractions (see page 165), but these are nothing to worry about.

Some safety issues, and circumstances when it's best to refrain from sex, are listed below. As always, if you have any questions speak to your GP.

When you should refrain from having sex
- If you experience bleeding. Most mild bleeding in pregnancy, especially during early pregnancy, is nothing to worry about, but if you do notice vaginal bleeding, refrain from intercourse until after you've been to your GP for a check-up.

- If you are at risk of pre-term labour, avoid having sex during the third trimester.

- Don't have sex once your waters have broken or if you are leaking amniotic fluid as there is a risk of infection.

- If you have cervical weakness (premature opening of the cervix) or placenta praevia (low-lying placenta – see page 183) follow your GP's advice on whether or not intercourse is safe for you.

- If your partner has genital herpes refrain from having vaginal or oral sex during an outbreak.

- Never blow up the vagina during sexual activity as it can cause a potentially fatal embolism.

- Anal sex is not recommended during pregnancy.

Your varying sex drive

You may find that your sex drive varies throughout your pregnancy. During the first trimester, with its rush of hormones and accompanying fatigue and nausea, you may want nothing more than a nice cup of tea and a good book at bedtime. But in the second trimester, some women report having the best sex of their lives. As well as extra lubrication, increased blood flow and high levels of hormones make your breasts and vagina more sensitive and readily aroused. It can be easier to reach orgasm, or even to have multiple orgasms, during this stage of pregnancy.

By the time the third trimester comes round and your pregnancy bump is large, just the physical discomfort and awkwardness you are experiencing can be a bit discouraging. So as your body changes through your pregnancy, you will find it necessary to adapt your sexual habits.

After 24 weeks you should avoid using the missionary position or any position that involves your partner pressing his weight on you. You may prefer to be on top as it allows you to control the speed and depth of penetration, but ultimately you know best what is comfortable and enjoyable for you at this stage of your pregnancy.

Recommended sexual positions for the later stages of pregnancy

- Kneeling/from behind: this position allows you to have sex without your bump getting in the way.

- Side by side: with your partner either behind or in front of you. Many women find deep penetration uncomfortable during pregnancy and this can be a gentler way to have intercourse.

- Sitting: your partner sits on a chair with you on top of him.

- If you want to lie down, shift yourself to the edge of the bed, where your partner can stand or kneel without pressing down on you.

If your partner is feeling rejected

During the first trimester and sometimes afterwards, nausea and exhaustion will probably mean that sex is actually the last thing on your mind. There is a risk that your partner might interpret this as rejection or evidence that, as he feared, you are drifting away from him. For this reason it's very important to talk to him about what you are feeling and explain to him that this won't be a permanent change.

It might also comfort your partner to know that during the second trimester, some women find that they feel more aroused than usual, so there's every chance you'll be making up for lost time later. As your pregnancy progresses further, you may find that you go off sex again because you are conscious of your changing body or are worried that sex might affect your baby. It is important to explain this to your partner, and remember that you may find that he is attracted to your new soft curves.

Other ways of showing affection

During any 'dry spells' it's also important to remember that there are many ways, apart from sex, in which you can show affection for each other. Stroking, cuddling, kissing and holding hands are great ways to maintain feelings of closeness. Don't be worried if some days you want almost constant cuddles and others you don't want to be touched at all – this is just another natural side effect of pregnancy hormones.

Explain to your partner that your hormones are affecting the way you are feeling, so that he is not bewildered by constant changes.

Smoking during pregnancy

It is important that you try to give up smoking during pregnancy. Remember that your smoking doesn't just affect you any more, it also affects your baby and it's important to be mindful of the fact that smoking during pregnancy is one of the most damaging things you can do to your unborn baby.

How smoking can affect your pregnancy

● Smoking damages your placenta, affecting the placental vessels and decreasing placental growth and blood flow.

- There is a greater risk of complications during pregnancy and labour, including higher rates of placental abruption, placenta praevia and bleeding during pregnancy. Smokers are five times more likely to develop eclampsia (see page 192) than non-smokers.

- Smoking stunts your baby's growth. Babies born to smokers tend to have lower birth weights. This is linked to problems in adult life such as diabetes and obesity. When you smoke you inhale carbon monoxide, which restricts the amount of oxygen your baby can receive. Oxygen is vital for their growth and development. Smoking not only restricts your baby's oxygen supply, but your baby's heart will beat faster as he tries to compensate for the lack.

- Smoking affects your baby's development. The babies of smokers are generally born smaller with less-developed organs, and smoking during pregnancy is also associated with a variety of other birth defects, including cleft palate. There is also evidence that smoking can affect your baby's mental and behavioural development, with higher incidences of attention deficit hyperactivity disorder (ADHD), hyperactivity and reduced attention spans.

- Smoking causes breathing problems for babies at birth as well as childhood asthma and respiratory problems. Your baby could have smaller airways and airflow would be on average 20 per cent less than a baby born to a non-smoking mother.

- Smoking is linked to miscarriage, premature birth and stillbirth.

- Babies born to smokers are more prone to infection and they may cry more and be harder to settle. As they get older they will be at increased risk of chest and ear infections.

● Babies born to smokers are twice as likely to die from cot death. Smoking by other members of the family after the birth is also a factor in this.

There is plenty of support for you if you want to stop smoking. The NHS can provide helpful advice and a dedicated quitting smoking service. Go and see your GP or midwife and they will point you in the right direction. You can also discuss whether using nicotine replacement therapy, such as gums and patches, might be the right option for you. You can get these on prescription, which is free when you are pregnant.

Other options include: the charity QUIT, Alan Carr's Easyway clinics and programme, hypnosis, electronic cigarettes and homeopathic methods. If you can't quit completely, the next best thing is to try to cut down as much as you can.

Don't pay any attention to the urban myth that quitting smoking cold turkey when you are pregnant is stressful for your baby: it won't be! The baby won't experience nicotine withdrawal and he will be healthier from the moment you extinguish your last cigarette.

If you have a partner who smokes, or you live with someone who does, see whether you can get them to quit or at least go outside when they smoke. This is especially important once your baby is born as the effects of passive smoking on his lungs are highly detrimental to his health and a contributing factor to cot death.

Medicinal drugs during pregnancy

If you can, it's best to avoid all types of medication during pregnancy. Of course if you become ill you may not be able to avoid it and there will be times when you decide that it is necessary to take something. But check with your GP first.

If you are buying over-the-counter medicines, speak to the pharmacist first and tell them you are pregnant and how many months. If you are already on a prescription medication speak to your GP and check that it is still safe to keep taking it. Always tell your GP that you are pregnant if they are prescribing medication to you.

Over-the-counter medications

● **Antihistamine – hay fever/allergies**

Some oral antihistamines aren't recommended during pregnancy, especially during the later stages, so it's best to err on the side of caution. See if you can treat your hay fever effectively with eye drops or nasal sprays. If these don't seem to help, visit your GP and discuss the best course of treatment. You will be advised which medication is best for you at your stage of pregnancy, be it over-the-counter or prescription.

● **Travel sickness/nausea**

If you normally suffer from travel sickness, try a motion-sickness travel band. These are worn around the wrists and are reputed to be very effective. They are also recommended for general nausea and morning sickness. Certain over-the-counter travel medications are said to be safe during pregnancy, but ask the pharmacist before you purchase any.

- **Painkillers**
  - * **Aspirin**

    Even though aspirin is occasionally prescribed in pregnancy to prevent clotting and to lower the risk of pre-eclampsia (see page 191), the general recommendation is that you do NOT take it when you are pregnant. Although the occasional dose probably won't hurt you, regularly taking aspirin has been linked to various problems, including miscarriage in early pregnancy, so steer clear of taking it unless it is prescribed by your GP.

  - * **Ibuprofen**

    Ibuprofen and other non-steroidal anti-inflammatory drugs (NSAIDs) are not recommended during pregnancy. These drugs have been linked to an increased risk of miscarriage and developmental problems in the first trimester and can cause delayed labour and other difficulties later on.

  - * **Paracetamol**

    This is considered to be the safest option when it comes to over-the-counter pain medication during pregnancy.

- **Laxatives**

  It is normal to experience constipation when you are pregnant. You are best advised to try to deal with the situation by increasing the amount of fibre you are receiving either in your diet or by taking a fibre supplement. If this doesn't help, speak to your GP before using a laxative.

- **Decongestants**

  Do not take decongestants that contain pseudoephedrine and phenylephrine and avoid taking cold medications that contain alcohol or cough medicine that contains codeine.

Natural and homeopathic remedies

Natural, homeopathic remedies and alternative therapies such as acupuncture can be very helpful during pregnancy. However, certain remedies and treatments are not to be recommended. For example, it is probably safest to avoid taking herbal medications during the first trimester in the same way that you would avoid pharmaceutical medications. If you are interested in complementary therapies and would like to use any remedies or treatments, make sure that you take advice from a fully qualified and trusted practitioner and don't forget to tell them that you are pregnant.

Recreational drugs

Taking recreational drugs when you are pregnant is to be avoided at all costs.

- **Cannabis**
  Cannabis use in pregnancy has been linked with miscarriage and low birth weight. And if you smoke it mixed with tobacco, then you are getting the detrimental effects of the tobacco as well.

- **Ecstasy, speed and other amphetamines**
  As well as miscarriage, premature birth and low birth weight, the use of amphetamines in pregnancy has been linked to placental complications including placental abruption. If you take speed during your pregnancy, especially during early pregnancy, your baby is at a higher risk of suffering from heart abnormalities, cleft palate, eye problems, a smaller head size and limb defects. There has been less research into the effects of Ecstasy in pregnancy

than into other illegal substances. However, much of what is sold as Ecstasy contains high levels of amphetamine, ketamine and other substances, so taking Ecstasy puts your baby at risk in the same way.

● LSD

LSD use carries a risk of miscarriage and chromosomal damage.

● Cocaine

Cocaine use in pregnancy has devastating effects. In the short term, it can cause your baby to suffer a stroke in the womb, possibly resulting in brain damage or death. Other effects include: placental abruption and placental complications, premature birth, low birth weight, small head size, urinary tract defects and heart defects.

In the long term, cocaine use in pregnancy has been linked to problems with cognitive function, learning and behavioural difficulties and problems with attention span.

● Heroin

Heroin use in pregnancy has serious consequences for your unborn baby. Babies born to mothers who use heroin share their addiction and have to be weaned off the drug after birth, when they can suffer from serious ill health, particularly associated with breathing. They are more likely to be born prematurely and have a low birth weight, and are at increased risk of stillbirth and having developmental and behavioural problems later in life. Babies born to heroin users are also much more likely to die of cot death. If you are addicted to heroin and discover that you are pregnant you should not attempt to come off it without speaking to your GP. Sudden withdrawal can result in miscarriage.

Getting support when things are difficult

Unfortunately some women have to deal with difficult emotional and domestic issues during pregnancy.

Domestic abuse affects many women and studies show that 30 per cent of all abuse starts during pregnancy (a NHS statistic) and existing abuse can also escalate during this time. If this is happening to you, please seek help, whether or not you're pregnant. The National Domestic Violence helpline (0808 2000 247) is confidential and open 24 hours a day (see Resources, page 332).

Domestic abuse isn't the only difficulty women might face during pregnancy. There can also be problems related to drugs and alcohol, emotional issues and mental health issues that need to be dealt with before the baby is born. By its very nature the emotional and life-changing aspects of pregnancy can bring these sorts of issues to the fore, for women and their partners. However, it is possible to get help. If you have problems with alcohol or drug dependency, or are suffering from emotional or mental health issues, please see our Resources section (pages 330–2).

5

Exercise During Pregnancy

Exercising in pregnancy is good for both you and your baby and will help you prepare, mentally and physically, for the challenges of birth and looking after a newborn baby. Try not to look on exercising as a chore, but rather as a chance to take a little me-time and look after yourself. It can bring a number of bonuses:

Exercise can help:

- The feel-good factor. Exercise makes you feel better: happier, stronger and more relaxed. When you exercise, your body releases endorphins, which are responsible for the rush of well-being you experience. Other hormones leave you feeling relaxed. It is a winning combination. The good news is that your baby also benefits as these hormones cross the placenta, leaving him happier and more relaxed too.

- Energy levels. Regular exercise has been found to boost energy levels, which is good when you are pregnant as you are very likely to be feeling far more fatigued than normal.

- Sleep. Sleep problems are common during pregnancy (see page 72). Studies have found that you will get to sleep better at night if you've exercised during the day. However, don't exercise just before you go to bed, as this might have the effect of stimulating you and keeping you awake instead.

● Labour. Exercising in pregnancy will help you become fitter and prepare you for labour. Although there is no way of predicting exactly how your labour will go, and you should never feel guilty or at fault if you have a problematic labour, it has been shown that being physically fit and staying active during pregnancy makes childbirth easier to cope with.

● Getting back into shape after your baby's birth. If you keep fit during your pregnancy you should regain your pre-baby shape more quickly and easily after the birth. Exercise can help keep you within the recommended healthy range of pregnancy weight gain (see page 37).

● Circulation. Exercise keeps your circulation going and your blood flowing. This is particularly important during pregnancy and can help you with common pregnancy issues such as restless leg syndrome (see page 75), cramps (see page 76) and swollen ankles (see page 154). Increased circulation also benefits your baby as he will be receiving more oxygenated blood to help with his growth and development.

● Backache. Keeping fit and strong during pregnancy should help your body, and more specifically your back, cope with the demands being placed on it by the extra weight you are carrying.

● Constipation. This is another of those common pregnancy niggles, but moderate activity and exercise encourage bowel movements and should help get a sluggish system going. Just a 10-minute walk around the block can do the trick.

Pelvic floor exercises

Whatever type of exercise you favour during pregnancy, it is very important to do your pelvic floor exercises before, during and after pregnancy. The National Institute for Health and Clinical Excellence (NICE) recommends that all women should do pelvic floor exercises and particularly during their first pregnancy. These exercises reduce your risk of stress incontinence after your child is born as well as helping with your labour and delivery.

The pelvic floor is a sheet of muscles, connective tissue and ligaments stretching from the pubic bone at the front to the back of the spine. They support the uterus, bowel and bladder. When your pelvic floor becomes weak with ageing and after childbirth, you may experience pelvic floor problems such as incontinence and prolapse. About one-third of women get urinary stress incontinence and one in 10 get faecal incontinence after the delivery. Do your pelvic floor exercises whenever you think about it and have the chance – at least 10 times per day. It may help to imagine that you have a string attached to these muscles that passes right through your body and comes out at the top of your head. Imagine you are gradually pulling up on this string.

Sitting down with your eyes closed, visualise the pelvic floor muscles, which hold your bladder and uterus in place.

Pull these muscles in and up, holding while you count to five. Release.

How to exercise in pregnancy

Exercising in pregnancy doesn't have to mean hitting the gym or going to a class if that doesn't suit you. Just incorporating 30 minutes of low-impact exercise into your everyday life is enough to make a difference and feel the benefits. Those 30 minutes don't

A word of warning

When contemplating taking exercise during pregnancy, it is better to do some regular gentle exercise rather than opting for something taxing that you only do once a fortnight. You are aiming to keep your body in shape and improve your stamina rather than pushing yourself to the limit so that you end up feeling exhausted and can't face exercising again for a while afterwards.

Exercise is not recommended if you suffer from:

- Placenta praevia.
- Pre-eclampsia.
- Incompetent cervix.
- History of recurrent miscarriages.
- High blood pressure.
- Pre-existing heart and lung conditions.
- Vaginal bleeding.
- Multiple pregnancies – extra caution should be taken if you are expecting twins. If you are carrying three or more babies, you need to be extremely careful about exercising.
- Anaemia – this only applies to severe cases. Speak to your GP and follow their advice.
- Gestational diabetes.

even have to be consecutive, so if you can manage a 15-minute walk to the bus stop, 10 minutes of stretching in front of the TV and a bit of gardening that will be plenty.

The key with exercise is to be consistent, and to be sensible: it's better to do a little moderate exercise every day rather than going all out once or twice a week and doing nothing in between.

If you weren't active or into keeping fit before you became pregnant, it is important that you don't suddenly throw yourself into an over-strenuous regime. Be kind to yourself. Aim for three 30-minute sessions of moderate exercise a week and slowly build up. Think of warming up and cooling down as being part of your exercise regime.

If you were a regular at the gym pre-pregnancy, be aware that you will probably have to adapt or modify your routine, especially by the time you get to the third trimester of pregnancy. This isn't the time to be setting personal bests, so don't push yourself too hard – it won't benefit you or your baby. However, that doesn't mean that you can't exercise until you feel satisfied, it just means you might have to vary your routine to achieve your goals.

Take care with exercise

When you are taking any form of exercise during pregnancy, you need to be careful not to overdo it, and this is particularly true if the weather is hot. If you are going to an exercise class, tell the teacher that you are pregnant and how many weeks you are, in case there are particular exercises that it might be best to avoid.

- If you suddenly feel dizzy or nauseous, stop straight away rather than pushing yourself to carry on. If you experience any vaginal bleeding or pains in your stomach, if you faint or your vision gets blurry, then you should seek medical advice immediately.

- It is important to warm up properly before taking exercise. That way your body will be prepared for the workout. Get a light sweat going with five to ten minutes of light to moderate activity. Cooling down involves doing the same activity again. Be sure to check that the activity you choose is appropriate and safe for your stage of pregnancy (see below).

- Keep a bottle of water nearby, taking care to drink small, frequent sips and to make sure that you don't let yourself get dehydrated.

- Don't exercise immediately after eating a large meal – it's generally suggested that you allow as much as four hours between eating a meal and taking exercise. If you need regular snacks, don't worry – it is fine to eat something light, such as soup or toast, a couple of hours before exercising.

Choosing the right type of exercise

Which type of exercise is best for you during pregnancy? There are some forms that are particularly suited to pregnant women, some that can be done in moderation or with modifications and others that are best avoided altogether.

Warning

If you aren't sure about any sport, check with your GP or midwife, and always talk to them before embarking on any kind of new fitness regime.

Ideal exercises during pregnancy

These exercises are low impact and as such are ideal to undertake during pregnancy. As with everything, moderation is key, so take care not to overdo it!

Walking

Walking is the simplest and easiest form of exercise. It is free, doesn't require any special equipment (though a good pair of comfy trainers will help), it can be done anywhere, at any time, and it is suitable right through to the end of your pregnancy.

Walking can be incorporated into your daily routine – walking to work or to the shops rather than hopping into the car or taking the bus. You can combine it with exercising the dog or you can get off the bus a stop early and walk the rest of the way. Walking can be wonderfully refreshing, mentally and physically, so just try walking for walking's sake.

Many people find that a brisk walk in the middle of the day helps their concentration and creativity and as so many of us are leading sedentary indoor lifestyles, getting out of the house can re-energise you and leave you feeling calmer all round.

If you can, try to fit in a couple of dedicated walks each week. If these can be done in inspiring surroundings – the local countryside, a particularly charming inner-city park or an inspiring part of town – so much the better.

Yoga

Yoga can be a real benefit during pregnancy and it can help you get through these months with the least discomfort, keeping you healthy in mind and body. Your flexibility will be enhanced, allowing you to adapt to different positions in labour, and more elastic ligaments will help reduce pain in labour. Yoga means 'union' and the emphasis it places on the mind–body connection seems particularly apt for this transformative time of your life, when awareness of your body is heightened. Yoga strengthens, stretches and relaxes your body, assisting focus and awareness. It teaches you about the importance of breathing and how it can be used to assist you physically and mentally.

It is important that you find a dedicated yoga-for-pregnancy class taught by a qualified teacher. Modified yoga positions will be taught so that you can be certain you aren't doing anything that might harm your baby or cause injury to your already loosened joints. These classes will also be focused on exercises and breathing techniques that will help you prepare for childbirth.

If you do attend a regular yoga class make sure it is a relatively slow-paced Hatha or Iyengar class and be sure to tell the instructor that you are pregnant, even if you are not yet showing. Avoid energetic, dynamic styles, such as Ashtanga, and some fast-paced Hatha classes. They require real physical exertion. Some make you sweat a great deal, which is to be avoided during pregnancy.

You should not attend Bikram yoga sessions, which are carried out in a heated room, for the same reasons that you shouldn't sauna or steam when pregnant. Overheating can be dangerous for your baby.

It is recommended that you wait until after your first trimester before you begin pregnancy yoga classes.

Swimming

Swimming is a great exercise for pregnancy because the water supports your extra weight. This is pleasant for you as you get the relief of feeling lighter, if only temporarily. It also makes exercising easy on your joints, which can be put under strain when you are pregnant.

There are a variety of aqua-aerobics-style classes you can try, some of which are designed specifically for pregnant women. Check your gym or local swimming pool and see what is available. You can do swimming and water-based exercise right up to the end of your pregnancy.

Pilates

Pilates can be highly beneficial during pregnancy because it works the core muscles and strengthens the tummy, pelvic floor and back muscles, which are key for helping you achieve good posture, balance and strength. This is particularly useful because of all the extra strain you will be feeling on your back during pregnancy. The stronger your core and abdominal muscles are, the better your back will cope. Pilates is also calm and relaxing and a good way of toning and strengthening without getting out of breath and sweaty.

Make sure that you go to a Pilates class that is specifically geared towards pregnancy as it is very easy to damage the stomach muscles during pregnancy (which is why you shouldn't do sit-ups) and with many Pilates exercises focusing on this area you want to make sure you aren't doing anything that could cause you problems.

Take care with these exercises

The following exercises can be undertaken with some caution:

Running

If you aren't already a runner, you should not take it up for the first time during pregnancy. Running and jogging can put a lot of pressure on your joints and ligaments and as your size increases this pressure will increase.

If you love to run, try to modify your routine so that you are not pushing yourself as hard and fast as you might do normally, maintain a moderate pace and be sure not to get out of breath, overheat or become dehydrated.

Gym exercise machines

Most exercise machines are fine to use during pregnancy. Talk to your trainer or to a member of staff about what machines are suitable to use during pregnancy and which aren't. For example, the rowing machine is not advisable because of the danger of causing lower-back injuries, and power plates, which are now very popular, haven't been tested for safety during pregnancy. A staff member or trainer should also be able to advise you on how to modify what you are doing to prevent injury.

Weights

Lifting heavy weights is not advisable at any time during pregnancy, but do take advice from your GP on all weight lifting. If light weights have been part of your pre-pregnancy routine, it may be possible to continue, provided you take the appropriate medical advice. However, from the second trimester onwards you shouldn't lift weights while you are standing up. GPs recommend that you don't use hand weights that are much heavier than 1 kg (2 lb) due to the risk of hurting your back. Make sure, if you are lifting weights, that there is no possibility of dropping the weights on yourself, specifically on your stomach, so you must not lift weights while you are lying down, even at the beginning of pregnancy.

Cycling

Cycling is not recommended after the second trimester, due to the risk of being knocked off or falling off your bike and suffering an impact that could harm your baby. As your bump grows you may find balancing harder. However, using the exercise bike at the gym is absolutely fine.

Exercises to avoid

The following forms of exercise are off-limits during pregnancy:

Sit-ups

These may be fine during the early stages of pregnancy, but they will become more and more difficult as your abdomen expands. In any event, they are not advisable after four months of pregnancy has gone by. Lying on your back is uncomfortable anyway once you are past four months and, as your bump gets larger, you are at risk of causing damage to your stomach muscles. If you want to keep your abdominals strong during pregnancy try pregnancy Pilates instead.

Contact sports

Sports such as judo, karate, wrestling, fencing, rugby or any sport that might involve you being hit in the stomach should be avoided at all costs.

Ball sports

You should seek medical advice before contemplating playing sports such as football, cricket, netball, squash and tennis. You should avoid any ball game where a ball travels at a high velocity – it is a risk to your baby. Running around the court or pitch when you are heavily pregnant and your balance is off-kilter could result in a damaging fall or back injury.

If you love, and are experienced at, a sport such as tennis and you can't bear to give it up, use your judgement and take medical advice as to how long you are able to keep playing during pregnancy. Bear in mind the guidelines about overheating and overexertion in pregnancy.

Skiing, snow-boarding, horse-riding

You should avoid any sport where you risk falling over or falling off something at high speed. Extreme sports such as bungee-jumping or parachuting are also to be avoided.

Backpacking

The recommendation is that you don't exercise, walk or trek while carrying a heavy backpack as you risk damaging your back.

Scuba-diving

You shouldn't scuba-dive while you are pregnant because there could be problems with your baby decompressing. Studies have linked women scuba-diving in pregnancy with birth defects and premature birth.

Pregnancy exercise dos and don'ts

- DO be sure to include a variety of exercises so you don't get bored.
- DO use the right kit – sports bra, trainers and comfortable clothes that are breathable and stretchy.
- DO make sure that you tell your trainer or instructor that you are pregnant, even if you aren't showing yet.
- DO stay hydrated. Always take a bottle of water with you and keep sipping it.
- DO take a light healthy snack, such as a muesli bar, with you when you exercise, in case you feel faint or light-headed.
- DO take the time to warm up, cool down and do plenty of stretches. You are far less likely to injure yourself and it's important to give your body the time to adjust to being active.
- DO take extra care. When you are pregnant you release hormones that loosen your joints and ligaments to help your body adapt to its changing shape and make the birth easier. These same loose joints and ligaments mean that it is much easier to injure yourself.
- DO remember that your balance and co-ordination are going to be affected by your changing shape.
- DO listen to your body – stop if you feel dizzy or faint, if you feel pain or find yourself short of breath.
- DON'T overheat, it can be damaging for your baby, especially in the first trimester.
- DON'T push yourself too hard – you should expect to get tired more easily when you are pregnant, so go gently and stay within your comfort zone.
- DON'T exercise for too long each session. Exercising too hard in pregnancy has been linked to low birth weight in babies.

- DON'T get too heavily out of breath – you want to make sure you have enough oxygen for you and your baby. If you are struggling to talk while exercising, you are exercising too hard.
- DON'T let your heart rate get too high – once it's past a certain point your baby's will be raised too.

6

Your Antenatal Care

Discussing your antenatal care

Once you have carried out a home pregnancy test and received a positive result, you can make your first appointment with your GP. You can do this at any time to discuss your pregnancy and to start planning your antenatal care. At this early stage, your GP may give you information and advice and arrange a date for your booking appointment (see overleaf). Antenatal care is important as it allows your GP or midwife to monitor you and your baby – making sure that everything is going well. If you need any special attention, it can be picked up and addressed without delay. It can also help to predict any potential problems, answer any questions you might have and give you the chance to get to know the people who will be looking after you.

You can expect a certain amount of choice about where you go for antenatal care and who looks after you. This means that it is possible to have care near to where you live and even at home, making it easier for you to keep appointments. NICE (the National Institute for Health and Clinical Excellence) recommends that your first appointment should take place before 12 weeks and that it is a double appointment since there is a lot of information for you to take on board.

Your booking appointment

This appointment usually takes place some time between eight and twelve weeks of pregnancy. It may be carried out at your GP's surgery, at hospital, at a health centre or even at home. It is a long and thorough appointment with your GP or midwife, where you will have plenty of time to ask questions and to discuss any niggling worries or concerns that you may have. You will be given lots of advice and information about keeping healthy during pregnancy, including tips on diet and lifestyle. It can be useful to jot down any questions you have beforehand so that you don't forget anything once you are there.

You will also be told about the antenatal care you will receive during your pregnancy and the antenatal screening tests you will have to make sure that everything is fine with your baby (see page 112 for more on this). You will be given information about maternity and paternity benefits too (see page 263). Your GP or midwife will want to get a good picture of your general health and well-being and of your medical history, so it is important to answer questions honestly and to mention anything that you feel may be relevant. Although it may seem very early to be thinking about the birth itself, there will usually be some discussion about this, to allow you to consider your options and to think about your preferences in good time.

The specific areas that should be covered in the booking appointment include:

- The first day of your last period and your expected date of delivery (this can be calculated, provided that you have a regular cycle – see page 25).

- You and your partner's age and occupations.

- You and your partner's family history – so that you can identify any genetic diseases (see page 22).

- Any past pregnancies and their outcomes.

- Previous live births you may have had and if there were any complications associated with their delivery.

- Your general health, previous operations or medical illnesses.

- Recent cervical smears you have had and any surgery on the cervix.

- Drug allergies and recreational drug use.

- Your diet.

- Any history of domestic violence or sexual abuse.

- Smoking and alcohol intake.

- Your exercise regime.

A general examination will be carried out and during this the GP or midwife will want to record some of your medical information including:

- Your height and weight to calculate your BMI (see page 37). This is to assess whether you are very underweight (with a BMI of less than 18) or overweight (with a BMI over 30).

- Your baseline blood pressure to ensure that there are no pre-existing blood pressure problems. Your blood pressure can sometimes rise or fall during pregnancy and it is important that it is checked regularly. Some women get pregnancy-related hypertension, or high blood pressure. If you have high blood pressure it is important that it is checked regularly as some women can develop pre-eclampsia, a condition that may affect your health and your baby's health too. (For more on high blood pressure and pre-eclampsia, see page 191)

● Abdominal examination to check that your uterus feels the right size according to your dates – at 12 weeks it can just be felt. Your midwife or GP may be able to hear your baby's heartbeat at this appointment, though this isn't always possible as the baby is so small.

● Chest and heart examination – to ensure that you do not have an irregular heartbeat, breathing problems or heart murmurs.

An internal pelvic examination or breast examination is not usually carried out during this appointment. If your cervical smear is out of date (in other words, if you last had one more than three years ago), you will not be offered another until at least three months after you have had your baby.

A urine sample will usually be taken at this appointment, to make sure that you don't have any infection, and you will have a blood test to check for:

● Anaemia. A full blood count (FBC) will be taken, which gives your haemoglobin level. A low level of haemoglobin indicates that you may be anaemic. If you are anaemic, you are likely to feel very tired and will probably be given some form of iron supplement to ensure that your health and your baby's are not at risk. It is a good idea to make sure that you are eating plenty of foods that are rich in iron, such as red meat, fish, poultry, green leafy vegetables, wholegrain bread, pulses and dried fruit.

- Blood group and rhesus status. If you are rhesus negative you may produce antibodies after the birth of your baby if the baby is rhesus positive, which could lead to problems in a future pregnancy (rhesus disease – see page 206). Your GP or midwife will explain this and discuss the injections you can be given to prevent any risks.

- Hepatitis B.

- Rubella immunity status.

- Syphilis.

- HIV (you can opt out of this test if you want).

- Sickle cell anaemia and thalassaemia. Women from certain ethnic groups have a higher risk of suffering from these diseases and screening is recommended.

Armed with this information your GP or midwife will be able to see whether there are any problems that could suggest that your pregnancy is higher risk. Most women are cared for by their GP or midwife, but if there are indications that your pregnancy could be high risk, a hospital appointment will be made for you so that you can see the obstetric team and your care will be shared between the hospital and your GP or midwife.

If you require hospital care it may be because you have any of the following:

- Previous complications in pregnancy such as stillbirth, a small baby, high blood pressure, Caesarean section, pre-term labour, miscarriage.

- Heart disease, high blood pressure.

- Chronic lung diseases such as asthma.

- Diabetes and other endocrine diseases.

- Kidney disease.

- Blood disorders such as sickle cell anaemia, clotting problems, haemophilia.

- Neurological illnesses such as epilepsy.

- Psychiatric illnesses.

- Chronic viral infections – hepatitis, HIV.

- Regular drug or alcohol misuse.

- Cancer.

- Having a very low (under 18) or high (over 30) BMI (see page 37).

- Rhesus disease of the baby.

- Age – if you are over 40 or a teenager.

After the booking appointment your GP or midwife can identify any special care that you may require. This will include lifestyle advice such as:

- Stopping smoking (see page 83).

- Help with alcohol and drug misuse (see pages 51 and 88).

- Support for domestic violence (see page 90).

- Healthy eating, foods to avoid and safe food preparation (see Chapter 3).

- Exercise (see Chapter 5).

Supplements

At the booking visit, your GP or midwife may also discuss any supplements that you should be taking. Iron supplements are not generally given unless you are found to be anaemic, but you should be taking 400 micrograms a day of folic acid (see page 18). If you are epileptic, diabetic, suffer from coeliac disease or have a previous affected child this should rise to a dose of 500 micrograms a day. It is now recommended that pregnant women take vitamin D supplements – see page 46 for more on this.

Maternity records

All the information that is taken during your antenatal appointments is recorded in the 'maternity record book'. This is a record that you keep with you and take to each appointment. Many maternity units use a standardised national maternity record book, which collates all the information.

Your plan for care in pregnancy and delivery can be written in this book, which helps to decide what type of delivery will suit you best and also where best you should have your baby (at home, at a midwife-led birth unit or in hospital – see page 122).

The results of all your blood tests and scans can be added to your maternity record book. This will help any other doctor look after you, should you have an emergency and need to go to a different hospital at any point.

You should carry your maternity notes with you at all times at the later stages of pregnancy in case you go into labour suddenly – or need emergency care.

How many antenatal appointments?

If this is your first baby and there are no complications during your pregnancy, you will usually have ten appointments with your GP or midwife during your pregnancy. If you have already had a baby before this one and are considered low-risk, just seven appointments will usually be necessary. If you have any particular worries or concerns during your pregnancy and have a long wait before your next scheduled check, you can always go to see your GP before your next appointment is due.

Ultrasound scans

Ultrasound scans use sound waves rather than X-rays and are perfectly safe to have during pregnancy. An ultrasound scan allows a detailed assessment of the baby from early to late pregnancy and is not usually uncomfortable.

You may be offered two scans: one at around 12 weeks (first scan) and another around 18–20 weeks (anomaly scan).

The first scan

The first scan is done very early in your pregnancy to check that everything is going well. If you've had fertility treatment in order to get pregnant, if there have been problems with bleeding or pain or if you are unsure about your dates, this may apply to you. The scan may also be used to check whether you are expecting more than one baby. Very early scans are usually done by inserting the ultrasound probe into your vagina, so that the scanner is closer to the womb and can receive a better image of the baby.

The foetal heartbeat can normally be seen from about six weeks of pregnancy onwards.

Most women have their first scan towards the end of the first 12 weeks to see how the baby is growing and to check the heartbeat. This scan may also be done as part of a screening test for Down's syndrome (see nuchal scan, overleaf) and it may be accompanied by a blood test. The scan is usually carried out by placing a probe covered in ultrasound jelly over your abdomen. You will be asked to come to the appointment with a full bladder when you have the scan – though uncomfortable, this will help to make the ultrasound images clearer.

Second scan (anomaly scan)

A second scan is usually done at 18–20 weeks to check if there are any problems, or 'anomalies', with the baby, such as heart defects and problems with the spinal cord (spina bifida). You will be able to see quite a clear image of your baby on the screen, although you may need help from the sonographer (see page 121) in identifying how he is lying in your womb. His bones are displayed in white, while the rest of his body is displayed in grey. The sonographer will measure your baby and check that his organs all seem normal. They will also look at the placenta to make sure that it is lying in the right position, and will check that the amniotic fluid and umbilical cord look healthy.

Other scans

There are also extra scans that might be recommended by your doctor if you have any health concerns:

- If you are at high risk of pre-eclampsia, or have had this before or a small baby, you may be offered a scan of the blood flow to the uterus (a 'uterine artery doppler scan'). If this shows that the blood flow is reduced then aspirin may be given early on in pregnancy to reduce the risk.

- If you have had a previous early delivery or late miscarriage you may be offered a scan of the cervix to check that it is not opening and shortening prematurely. If the scan highlights problems, your doctor may discuss the need for a cervical stitch.

- If there is any discrepancy between the size of your uterus and your dates, or if you have had a previous small baby, then having growth scans through your pregnancy might be suggested to check the baby is growing well. If you have a twin pregnancy, growth scans will be booked every two to four weeks.

Tests for genetic abnormalities

Nuchal scan

A nuchal scan is a screening test for Down's syndrome, where the amount of fluid at the back of the baby's neck is measured. Babies who have Down's syndrome usually have more fluid than normal and a thicker area around the nape of the neck (the nuchal area). This test is carried out between 11 and 13 weeks of pregnancy. It is important to be aware that these tests don't give definitive answers about the baby having Down's syndrome, but give an estimate of your risk. Having a higher risk does not necessarily mean that your baby has Down's syndrome, and if you fall into a high-risk category you will be offered further tests.

Chorionic villus sampling (CVS) and amniocentesis

A CVS can be carried out between 10 to 13 weeks of pregnancy. This involves taking a sample of the placenta and it can be done through the neck of the womb or cervix. CVS can show whether the baby has a number of conditions such as Down's syndrome, cystic fibrosis and sickle cell anaemia. The initial results can be received as quickly as within one week. Generally, it is a very accurate test, though it may have to be repeated if there is not a proper sample. There is a slightly increased risk of miscarriage – around 2 per cent – after having a CVS.

An amniocentesis involves taking a sample of the amniotic fluid that surrounds the baby in the womb. It can only be carried out after 15 weeks of pregnancy. This test has a risk of miscarriage of 1 per cent.

Private or NHS care

You have an automatic right to have your baby on the NHS in the UK and the care is free, but you might want to choose to go private, provided you can afford it or are covered by appropriate health insurance. Ask your GP for advice on private care if you are keen on this choice, or look online for local options. Although private care has unique strengths in allowing you to have a one-to-one relationship with your consultant, you may well be perfectly happy with the usually excellent care provided by the NHS. The advantage of the NHS is that there is a large on-call team present on site at all times as well as back-up services, such as intensive care units, for the very small proportion of mothers and babies who need them.

Considering private care

Private care, with a consultant obstetrician, can be expensive as you will pay for the hospital costs, the obstetrician and the anaesthetist, should you need one. If you are considering this option, make sure that you know what is included in the price – for instance, are blood tests and scans included and are there package prices? It is also important to be clear whether there are facilities for urgent or emergency care, should the need arise, where the baby would be treated and whether you and the baby might have to transfer to another (NHS) hospital if there were complications. Not all hospitals or consultants offer private care and you may need to change to an alternative hospital if there are no facilities for private care at your local hospital.

Independent midwife

An alternative form of one-to-one care may be to have an independent midwife. These tend to specialise in home births. An independent midwife will offer personal care throughout your pregnancy and birth, but she can refer you for scans, blood tests and any other specialist treatment within the NHS. An independent midwife may not be able to look after you in your local NHS unit and should you need to transfer there, your care will be taken over by the doctors and midwives on the unit.

Birthing centre

Another option you may want to consider is going to a birthing centre. Some of these operate within the NHS and may be attached to hospitals, while others are fully independent. They offer a more relaxed environment for giving birth and may have facilities for water births or complementary therapies that are not available in a more traditional hospital setting. If you opt to go to a birthing centre and there are any complications during the birth, you may need to transfer to an NHS hospital.

Planning the birth

You may be surprised to find that, quite early in your pregnancy, you are asked questions about the sort of birth you would like. You may not have given this much thought yet and the birth may still feel as though it's a long way off. However, it is important to start thinking about the birth reasonably early on in pregnancy, since if you decide you'd like an independent midwife or want to use a private birthing centre, you will need to book this well in advance. You may also want to start finding out more about the different choices you could make and what the consequences of these can be.

What are your choices?

The main decisions you will be asked to make are about where you would like to give birth and about pain relief. You may have very strong opinions on this and know exactly what you'd like. If you are less certain, talk to your midwife or GP, research subjects you'd like to know more about and talk to other women about their birth experiences. However, keep in mind that whatever kind of birth plan you draw up, labour can be unpredictable and circumstances often change. It is important to accept beforehand that although a birth plan sets out what you would like to happen in an ideal world, this may not be possible in reality. Therefore you should not feel disappointed if your baby's birth ends up being quite different to the birth you had envisaged when drawing up the plan.

Choosing the care you'd like

In recent years, the need for women to be allowed to choose how they will be cared for during pregnancy and where they want to give birth has been more widely recognised. One of the concerns often expressed by pregnant women is that they fail to receive continuity of care, that there is not enough information available and that they are unsure about who is responsible for what.

There has now been extensive research into all aspects of ante-natal care, to decide what interventions and appointments are of benefit and who is best placed to carry them out. In addition, there is now more focus on allowing women to choose where they deliver, so that the process can be 'de-medicalised' if possible – after all, birth is a normal part of life.

In order to understand the process there are various health professionals who may manage some of your pregnancy care.

Health professionals you may encounter

General practitioner (GP)
The GP, or your family doctor, is an important link between you and the hospital. They can provide emergency care, but also offer

continuity of care for your baby when he is born. Most pregnancy care is managed between your GP, midwife and the hospital and is called 'shared care'.

Midwife

Your midwife is a highly trained professional who cares for you during pregnancy, labour and the period after your baby's birth. She (or sometimes he) is also trained in looking after the newborn baby and in helping to establish feeding. Your midwife has a key role in helping you decide where and how you will give birth, and they will help you put together your birth plan (see page 128).

You are most likely to receive care during pregnancy and birth from a midwife who may be based in a hospital clinic, at a community centre or in a GP surgery. She (or he) can refer you on for advice if any complications arise during your pregnancy, but if everything runs smoothly and the pregnancy is normal, she will be able to look after you throughout.

When you are in labour, the same midwife will look after you wherever possible, though shift patterns may make this impossible. Once you have given birth, the community midwifery team will be informed and one of them will come and visit you and your baby at home, to make sure that you are both doing well. This is very convenient as they can also check any bleeding, remove stitches if necessary, make sure you have no infections and ensure that the baby is feeding well and putting on weight.

Obstetric team

The hospital obstetric team is composed of doctors of varying experience with a consultant obstetrician in charge. If your pregnancy and delivery is uncomplicated you will not usually see the obstetric team at all. If there are complications or if advice is needed, your GP or midwife can refer you to them. This usually happens in the hospital. Some women have most of their care managed by the consultant team, but this is not necessary unless you have a more complicated pregnancy than normal.

In labour the obstetrician assists your delivery if progress is slower than normal or the baby seems to be distressed. He or she can assess whether the baby is showing a normal heart-rate pattern and if needed they will be able to perform a forceps (see page 302), ventouse (see page 303) or Caesarean section delivery (see page 306). All the doctors on the labour ward are trained to be expert in these procedures and they have 24-hour additional back-up from a consultant at all times. Many units now have a consultant present on the labour ward for up to 60 hours a week.

The obstetric team is often supported by other doctors, such as doctors specialising in diabetes, haematologists (who manage blood disorders), neurologists and cardiologists, all of whom can help with any associated medical conditions.

Anaesthetist

This is a doctor who specialises in pain relief during labour. He or she is responsible for giving epidurals/spinal anaesthesia and in some circumstances, though only rarely, administering general anaesthesia. This doctor will generally not see you before your labour unless there are concerns regarding the type of anaesthetic you may need. If you have previously suffered from a bad reaction to an anaesthetic or your anaesthetic is likely to be difficult to administer, for example because of medical problems or because you are overweight, the anaesthetist may see you to discuss the type of anaesthesia you may be suitable for and what the risks may be.

Paediatrician

The paediatrician looks after the baby when he is born. Every hospital labour ward has 24-hour access to an emergency paediatrician should your baby develop problems with breathing after his delivery or if he needs close monitoring after birth. In some cases such babies may need to go to a special care baby unit (SCBU) for more intensive monitoring. This may be more likely if the baby is born earlier than expected (before 37 weeks).

Some women go into labour before their delivery date or may need to give birth earlier than expected. In these cases it is better to be in a hospital with a special care baby unit that can care for you and your baby properly. In some cases, this may not be your local hospital and you may have to be transferred to another that has the appropriate support. This does not happen very often and the team caring for you usually only suggests this if they feel that the baby's health may be compromised by not moving you. This move can be unexpected and distressing, but the most important issue is that your baby gets the right support at the right time, as the early hours of life can be crucial to his future.

Once you have had your baby, the paediatrician or midwife will perform the routine baby checks (see page 297) before you are discharged and give you any general advice you need.

Ultrasonographers

The scans you have in pregnancy are carried out by doctors or sonographers. They can perform the early dating, nuchal and anomaly scans (see pages 112–14). If there are any concerns, they will refer you to an obstetrician, who has particular expertise in this field.

Health visitors
Health visitors are based in the community and you will see them after you have had your baby, when they take over the role of looking after you both from the midwife. They will ensure that the baby gets all the necessary checks and vaccinations and will offer you all the advice you need in the early days of your baby's life – about feeding, general health and care.

Where you can have your baby

The choices for delivery are:

- Hospital.
- A midwife-led birth unit.
- Home.

You may have some idea of how you would like to deliver your baby, and where, and it is best that you talk this through with the antenatal team, who will try to accommodate your wishes. They will also consider what would be most appropriate for you. Broadly, in a hospital, there will be a full complement of medical staff, such as the on-call obstetric team and consultant, whereas in a midwife-led birth unit or at home, you will be looked after by a midwife.

The hospital

All hospitals run tours of their labour wards so that you can become familiar with the location of the labour ward in the hospital and know what it looks like. These tours are conducted by a midwife and you can ask questions on the spot. Even if you do not intend to have a hospital birth, it is worth knowing how to get to your local delivery unit just in case an emergency arises and you need to be seen urgently.

If you give birth in a hospital, the midwife will go through your birth plan with you when you arrive – even if you were originally intending to give birth at home.

Although some women feel that giving birth in a hospital 'medicalises' them too much (perhaps making it more likely that they will receive medical intervention), others prefer to have access to a doctor on site and other facilities such as high-dependency care, should the need arise.

If you choose to give birth in hospital and there aren't any complications, you can often be discharged and allowed to return home within four to six hours of having your baby.

What the labour ward tour consists of

- A description of all the staff you may encounter and what their area of expertise is – who will look after you and at what stage.

- Location of facilities such as the antenatal ward, delivery unit, postnatal ward and neonatal service and their visiting hours. (It's as well to be aware in advance that small children are generally not allowed to visit when you are a patient on the ward or when you are in labour – to reduce the risk of infection.)

- A view of a delivery room (if possible).

● Familiarisation of equipment used during the birth such as birthing balls and mats, TENS machines and birth pools.

Midwifery-led birth unit

These units may be located in the same building as the hospital
unit or they may be completely independent of the hospital. The
units are run by midwives and their function is to facilitate normal
births. Their advantage is that they often feel much more relaxed
and less busy than hospitals. You can be looked after by a midwife
you may already know well and that will give you a good feeling
of continuity. Many women have had very positive experiences in
having normal vaginal deliveries in what feels like a much more
natural environment. You can have access to simple pain relief in
labour, but not options such as an epidural, for which you need
an anaesthetist. Some birth units have a birthing pool available,
but it is worth confirming this beforehand if you think you might
want to use one.

Home births

Both the Royal College of Obstetricians and the Royal College
of Midwives support home births for women with uncomplicated pregnancies, yet only 2 per cent of women opt to have their
babies at home. A key advantage of a home birth is that you are
able to give birth in familiar surroundings and you do not need
to leave the comfort of your own home or even your family. In
the same way as in a midwifery-led birth unit, you will be looked
after by a midwife you may already know well.

Possible transfer to hospital

In both a midwifery-led birth unit and in a home birth, a small
proportion of women need to transfer to hospital if things aren't

going as well as expected. Reasons for this may include poor progress in labour, breathing problems in the baby, the need for epidural pain relief and maternal bleeding. When you are thinking about where you'd like to have your baby, you should consider how easy it might be to transfer to hospital when you're actually in labour, if this became necessary, and whether there are any local circumstances that may delay this. Transfers to hospital can be stressful and do carry a risk if the hospital is some distance away. This is why some women choose to be in midwife-led birth units that are attached to a hospital.

Reducing transfer risk

A good way to reduce your chances of needing a transfer to hospital during labour is to check whether you fit the criteria for a low-risk pregnancy and delivery. However, if you are a first-time mother it is very hard to define what risk category you fall into as it is difficult to predict how your baby's birth may progress. Unsurprisingly, more first-time mothers have to be transferred during labour than mothers who have already had a baby. If you have already had a baby without any problems, you may well be an ideal candidate for a home birth or a midwife-led unit.

Criteria for non-hospital births

Each hospital has criteria for those they consider able to have a baby outside the hospital. You will be able to discuss these with your midwife, who will be able to tell you whether you would be considered to be putting yourself and your baby at risk by opting to give birth outside the hospital.

Pain relief

One of the things you need to think carefully about is what sort of pain relief you might prefer to use in labour. It is good to think about this well ahead of time when you are compiling your birth plan. It is hard to know in advance how you might feel about dealing with labour once it happens, especially if this is your first baby. However, it's still a good idea to have thought through the different options available and to have considered what you might prefer if you need it. It's important to remember that we all have different pain thresholds, so what might be acceptable pain to you may be unacceptable to someone else and vice versa. For your pain relief options, see page 285.

What happens in antenatal classes?

Good preparation really pays off when you are thinking about labour, birth and looking after your baby afterwards. There are a number of good sources of information to help you plan and prepare. Antenatal classes cover a range of topics, giving information on pregnancy, birth, feeding your baby and a variety of parenting tips.

Topics covered include:

● Good nutrition.

● Keeping fit and healthy.

● Pelvic floor exercises.

- Making a birth plan.

- Labour.

- Different types of delivery.

- Pain relief and relaxation techniques.

- What to buy and how to prepare the nursery.

- Baby feeding – tips on breast- and bottle-feeding.

- Looking after yourself after delivery.

- Sex and contraception.

- Postnatal blues and depression.

Each hospital runs a course of antenatal classes to prepare you for delivery and afterwards, and you are strongly advised to sign up for one during the last trimester. These classes comprise groups of women who are often at the same stage as yourself and partners are encouraged to attend most of the sessions.

Making friends

You will probably find that you can make friends and build up a good support group of other women that you have met at these classes. It is often reassuring to see that other people have just as many questions about birth as you do. Information from these classes can really help you formulate your own birth plan and include your partner in vital decisions. The atmosphere is relaxed and informal and it is easy to ask questions. Classes are often held at the weekend or evenings to make them as convenient as possible if you are working.

Good support groups

As well as the hospital-run classes there are a number of other useful support groups.

- The best-known support group is the National Childbirth Trust (see Resources, page 328), which runs its own classes and has a useful website for tracking down further information. Their classes are usually given to small groups and there may be a fee.

- Pregnancy yoga classes are very useful for helping keep yourself as fit and healthy as possible and you can usually find them at local gyms or as private classes. Look online for convenient ones to join. (For more on this, see page 97.)

- You may be eligible to access the Sure Start Children's Centres, which provide support for mothers, babies and children under the age of five. These government initiatives work to help create the best environment for parents to bring up their children in terms of advice with parenting, nutrition and educational support (for further information, see www.direct.gov.uk).

Making your birth plan

At some point during the third trimester, your midwife will encourage you to make your birth plan. Your maternity notes have a dedicated space for these to be included, but additional sheets may be added if there are other things you want to include.

Your midwife and the antenatal classes are a good source of information to help you decide what you want to happen at the birth of your baby.

The birth plan covers issues such as:

● Where you would like to deliver.

● The type of pain relief you would prefer.

● How mobile you want to be during labour.

● Who you want to support you during labour.

● Whether you want to breast-feed your baby immediately after delivery.

● Whether you want skin-to-skin contact with your baby immediately after delivery.

It is important to be pragmatic when drawing up your birth plan because things may not necessarily go exactly the way you envisage. It would be unsafe to stick rigidly to the birth plan if it compromises your health or that of your baby. If this is your first baby, you don't know how you're going to react to the situation until you are actually going through it and it can be impossible to predict what may happen. Therefore it's best to keep an open mind, while forming a general idea about what you are aiming for – and for others to be aware of this too. That way you can avoid disappointments.

An example of a birth plan

Name:	Sarah Smith
DOB:	8th June 1987
UNIT No:	0592102

The following is a list of the preferences I have for the birth of my baby. I understand that these may change, depending on my experience in labour.

Place of birth:	Midwife unit, Montrose.
Birthing partner:	Husband, Ben Smith. To be with me at all times.
Type of birth:	I would like to be able to move around as I please during labour while wearing a TENS machine.
	I would like the opportunity to use a birthing ball, lots of pillows/bean bags and the birthing pool as pain relief for some of the first stage and possibly the second stage.
	I may also decide to use homeopathic remedies (particularly in the first stage).
Atmosphere:	I would appreciate that the lighting in the birthing room be kept low and that verbal contact be minimised to allow me to fully relax.
	I will bring CDs and massage oil for use by my birthing partner.
	I would prefer that the number of midwifery/ nursing personnel be kept to a minimum.

However, I am happy for one midwife/nursing student to be present.

Eating and drinking: I would like to be able to eat and drink as I wish during labour.

Pain relief: TENS machine or water, gas and air.

I would like the option of having pethidine/diamorphine if I feel I require it, and if there is likely to be sufficient time before delivery – I would appreciate some guidance on this from the midwife at the time.

Monitoring: Intermittent handheld monitoring of baby would be my preference.

I would prefer vaginal examinations to be kept to a minimum and only if absolutely necessary.

Intervention: Unless it is deemed essential for the health of the baby, I would prefer not to have any artificial acceleration of labour.

I would like my waters to break naturally.

I would like to avoid an episiotomy and I would rather tear naturally (unless it appears I am going to tear badly).

I would welcome instruction from the midwife regards pushing in the second stage.

Actual birth: I am keen to try to deliver in the pool if I am comfortable there.

I would like my baby handed to me as soon as possible for skin-to-skin contact.

I wish the midwife/nursing staff to cut the umbilical cord.

I would like my baby to be given an injection of vitamin K.

Third stage: I would like the option of delivering my placenta naturally, but I may change my mind! In my previous labour I requested an injection to speed up placental delivery.

Postnatal: I would appreciate advice regarding breast-feeding.

If my labour is uncomplicated and my baby is healthy on delivery I would prefer to be discharged as soon as possible.

Complications: I am aware that, should there be any complications (whether in labour, delivery, postnatal or with my baby's health), that we will require transfer to the nearest hospital. I would prefer this to be Aberdeen Maternity Hospital, as it is closer to my home.

Thank you for your consideration.

Choosing a birth partner

Having the right support during labour is important as it will help your labour and birth to run more smoothly. Research has shown that having the same midwife providing one-to-one care is linked with better birth outcomes, and having the right person with you as a birth partner can have the same effect.

When you are writing your birth plan, you should consider who you would like to be with you when you are in labour. It may be your partner, another relative, such as your mother or sister, or a close friend. Professional birthing assistants called 'doulas' are another option. The use of doulas has also been associated with good outcomes for delivery and fewer medical interventions.

PART 2

The Stages of Pregnancy

7

The First Trimester

This section of the book will guide you in your nine-month journey through pregnancy and will help you find out more about each step along the way. It will explain how your baby is growing each month, and discuss the changes you may be noticing in your own body as well as giving lots of helpful tips and advice.

Three trimesters

A pregnancy is divided into three trimesters, each covering a period of about three months. The first stage of pregnancy is known as the 'first trimester', and will take you right up to the end of the third month.

When is your pregnancy dated from?

Your pregnancy is dated from the first day of your last period, which can be rather confusing at first, as you don't conceive until the middle of your monthly cycle, about a fortnight after this. You will probably not find out that you are pregnant until the end of this first month, at the earliest, as missing a period is usually the first sign to look out for, though there are others, too, such as tender breasts. By the time your period is due, you will be four weeks pregnant if you have a regular menstrual cycle.

The first month

At the start of each menstrual cycle, a number of eggs begin to grow inside sacs, known as follicles, in the ovaries. One of the follicles will become dominant, growing bigger than the others, until eventually it is mature. Then the egg breaks out of the sac and travels down the fallopian tube towards the womb. At this stage, you are at your most fertile and the egg is ready to be fertilised by your partner's sperm. During sex, sperm are released into your vagina and travel up through your cervix to the fallopian tubes, towards the egg. The sperm can only survive for about 24 hours after being released. When the sperm meet the egg, just one of them will break through the outer layer, in order to fertilise it.

Once this happens, the fertilised egg (or embryo) begins to grow. It develops cells, which keep multiplying by dividing up until eventually, about five days after fertilisation, a cavity starts to appear in the centre. At this point, the embryo forms into a structure called a blastocyst, which is the next stage of development.At around a week or so after fertilisation, the lining of the uterus thickens and the blood supply increases, ready for the blastocyst to attach. As soon as the blastocyst has implanted into the womb lining, pregnancy hormones begin to circulate in the body. The blastocyst is still just a mass of cells at this point, but they begin to divide into layers, which will form the different parts of the baby's body and the placenta. At the end of this first month, the blastocyst is still very tiny and is no more than a millimetre long.

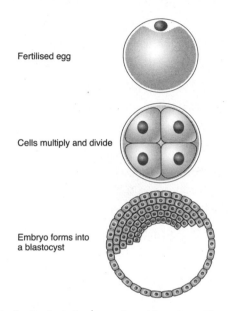

Fertilised egg

Cells multiply and divide

Embryo forms into a blastocyst

The fertilised egg develops cells and forms into a blastocyst

By this point, you will have raised levels of the pregnancy hormone human chorionic gonadotrophin (HCG), in your body and this can be detected in your urine when you do a home pregnancy test.

Once you have received a positive pregnancy test result, you should let your GP know, so that you can start to get the right antenatal care. You will be given a date for your first antenatal booking appointment with your GP or with a midwife. This isn't usually carried out until you are at least eight weeks pregnant and it will be a more lengthy appointment, where there will be plenty of time for you to ask questions. (See page 106 for more on this.)

The first month – changes in your body

During the first four weeks of your pregnancy there are often no signs that you are pregnant at all. You may be unaware that you are even pregnant at this stage, and it is perfectly normal not to have any indicators of the changes that are taking place in your body.

Implantation bleeding

Up to one-third of pregnant women may have some bleeding, known as 'implantation bleeding'. This may occur at around the time that you would have expected to have your period, so this can be misleading. The bleeding is usually rather scanty, more like spotting than a regular period, and is often intermittent, only lasting for a day or two. The discharge is often a light pink or brown colour.

Signs of pregnancy

Although many women don't have any sign of pregnancy at this very early stage, others say that they just 'know' they are pregnant straight away and there are some changes that it may be possible to spot even at this point. For example:

- Changes to your breasts. You may find that you have very tender or sensitive nipples, or they may tingle. Your breasts themselves may start to feel different, perhaps more full and heavy or a bit lumpy and sore.

- Nausea. Some women feel sick or nauseous very early in pregnancy. Although sickness in pregnancy is often called 'morning sickness', it can happen at any time of the day. Your nausea may be exacerbated by a heightened sense of smell, which can also occur during early pregnancy. (For more on nausea, see page 144.)

- More frequent urination. Pregnancy hormones can make you need to go to the loo more often, even in the very early days of pregnancy.

- Tiredness. You may find that you feel generally exhausted and lacking in energy.

- Changes to your sense of taste. Women sometimes go off certain foods during early pregnancy and a sudden aversion to coffee, wine or a particular food may be the first clue that you are pregnant. Increasing hormone levels can affect the make-up of your saliva and you may get an odd taste in your mouth in early pregnancy, which women often describe as 'metallic'.

The second month

You may not find out you are pregnant until the second month of pregnancy, and there won't be any outward signs that you are. However, there are huge changes going on inside your body and you are likely to begin to notice some signs of pregnancy yourself.

Telling other people
The decision about when to tell other people that you are expecting a baby may also arise during this month. As mentioned earlier on page 28, you may want to tell everyone that you are pregnant the moment you have a positive pregnancy test result, or you may prefer to wait until you've got through the first trimester, when

the chance of miscarriage is hugely diminished. Sometimes when you are feeling very tired and perhaps finding it hard to keep up your normal commitments, you may prefer to tell people rather than having to make excuses. How you feel about this is a very personal thing and there is no right or wrong way to deal with it.

The second month – your growing baby

Your baby changes very rapidly during this month. At four weeks, he still looks a bit like a miniature tadpole, but during the second month he will develop arms and legs and his heart will start beating. It will beat much more rapidly than yours and there may be fluctuations in the rate. If you have an ultrasound scan during this

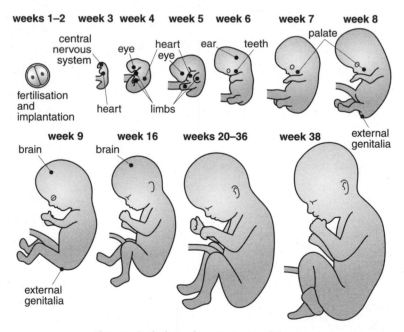

The growth of a foetus from week one to full term

month (see page 112), which you may do if there are any reasons for particular concern or if you have had fertility treatment, you should be able to see the baby's pulsing heartbeat by this point. If you have a scan and it shows a healthy heartbeat at this stage, it is a good indicator that things are looking positive for the rest of your pregnancy.

Early development

This early stage of development is very important as the structure of the baby's body and all the major organs are formed, even though the embryo is still only about 2.5 cm (1 in) long. The brain and the spinal cord are developing very rapidly and the baby's arms will be bent at the elbow and his fingers and toes will start to grow. The hands and arms develop more rapidly than feet and legs. The baby's facial features will also begin to appear in the second month, with eyes and a nose forming. The eyes are quite far apart at this stage of development and they are covered over, although the eyelids are forming. The ears are starting to grow, too, and the jaw and tiny tooth buds are developing. The baby's head is still very big in relation to the rest of his body and it curls over on to his chest. The skin will become quite downy as hair starts to grow.

The placenta and umbilical cord, which feed the baby, are also developing at this stage. The baby is using the nutrients you are providing to support this period of rapid growth and change, which is why it is important that you try to eat as healthily as you can. Folic acid plays a vital role during this time, so it's important to remember to take your folic acid supplements (see page 18).

Your baby will actually start moving about a bit at this stage, although it will be some time before you are able to feel these movements yourself.

The second month – changes in you

By the end of the second month, you are likely to have had some signs of pregnancy. Although there won't be any changes that are visible to other people, there are huge changes taking place inside your body and so it is hardly surprising if you start to feel more easily tired than usual. You may find that you feel exhausted by the end of the day and that you are longing for your bed. You may even feel a bit dizzy, lightheaded or faint at times.

Nausea

Another common sign during this early stage of pregnancy is sickness or nausea. Although we talk about 'morning sickness', it can occur at any time of day. You may just feel slightly nauseous and this is often triggered by certain smells as your sense of smell can become more acute at this time, or you may suffer bouts of quite severe vomiting. If you are feeling particularly rough, it may help to know that morning sickness usually eases and goes altogether as your pregnancy develops and most women feel much better by the second trimester. Hormonal changes in your body are thought to be responsible for making you feel sick, and it has been suggested that sickness may even be a good sign, demonstrating the body's defence mechanism working against ingesting toxins during pregnancy. Morning sickness doesn't have an adverse effect on your baby and it's only if you are so ill that you actually lose weight that it can affect the baby's weight. If your nausea is so bad that you are vomiting and cannot keep fluids down you will need to go to the hospital to be examined. You may need to stay in while you are given intravenous fluid and anti-sickness tablets until your nausea calms down.

What to do about morning sickness

If you are suffering from morning sickness, there are some things that may help:

- Eating small snacks throughout the day may keep nausea at bay more effectively than coping with three large 'main' meals.

- Having some plain food, such as a piece of dry toast or a cracker, every few hours will ensure that your stomach isn't empty, which seems to make sickness worse.

- Eating a couple of dry crackers in bed before you get up in the morning can help to circumvent morning sickness. Keep a supply by your bed at night, ready for when you wake up.

- Ginger is good for soothing feelings of sickness. You may want to try eating ginger biscuits or drinking ginger tea or ginger beer.

- Savoury snacks are often better for combating nausea than sweet things.

- Carbohydrates are good for tackling morning sickness (in the form of plain crackers, dry bread or toast).

- Acupressure wristbands, sold to combat travel sickness, can be helpful.

- If the smell of cooking makes you feel nauseous, you may want to try to eat more cold meals than usual.

- Some women find that sucking boiled sweets or lollipops works well.

- Getting more rest than usual can be helpful, and make sure you get plenty of sleep too.

- Ensure you keep hydrated – drink lots of fluids, but sip them slowly if you're feeling ill.

- Fatty or spicy foods can make your sickness feel worse, so it's probably best to avoid them.

- Getting plenty of fresh air and exercise can be beneficial.

- Making sudden, jerky movements can make your nausea worse, so moving about more calmly and slowly may help.

- A high-protein meal in the evening can be good as you will feel fuller for longer, which will stop you becoming nauseous.

- Some people recommend lemons in different guises – sipping tart lemonade or lemon juice in water, or even just sniffing lemons!

Indigestion

You may also find you suffer from some indigestion or heartburn, even at this early stage of pregnancy, so avoiding foods that seem to trigger this is a good idea. You may find it helpful to eat smaller, more frequent, meals to avoid indigestion.

Food cravings

Some women start to crave certain foods in early pregnancy, or to suddenly take a dislike to other things that they have always eaten happily before.

Other signs of pregnancy

You may need to urinate more frequently, and this is likely to continue throughout the pregnancy. Many women find that their breasts feel tender or swollen, and some notice changes in their skin too (see page 63). You may suffer from an outbreak of spots (see page 66) or your skin may feel drier than usual.

Vaginal discharge

During early pregnancy, women sometimes worry about increased vaginal discharge. This is quite normal as the changes in your body can lead to an increased watery discharge being produced. If the discharge is an odd colour or has an unpleasant smell, you should seek advice from your GP or midwife.

Aches and pains and cramping

You may feel concerned if you have any aches and pains or cramping during early pregnancy, however this can be very common as your womb is changing shape and growing, ready for your baby. Discuss it with your GP or midwife if you are worried, and seek medical advice immediately if you have severe cramps that are accompanied by bleeding.

Feeling emotional

You may feel more emotional, or even tearful, than usual and you may be worried about your baby and the pregnancy. It is only natural to be anxious, but if your fears become overwhelming talk to your GP about how you are feeling. Eating properly (see Chapter 3) and getting enough sleep can help you feel calmer, and taking some regular exercise (see Chapter 5) can be a real tonic if you are feeling down. Don't try to be 'superwoman', but rather take advantage of any opportunities you have to get a bit of a rest or take a nap. The chores can always wait until later. There are huge changes going on in your body and you need to be kind to yourself and be careful not to overdo things.

The third month

By now, you will probably be starting to grow more accustomed to being pregnant, and if you've been feeling very sick or tired, you are likely to begin to feel better soon as these symptoms generally fade towards the end of the third month. You will be gaining some weight by this stage, and will be noticing a change in your shape too. This is the final leg of the first trimester of pregnancy, and if you have been feeling anxious about the possibility of miscarriage, it will be reassuring to know that as you move into the second trimester the risk is significantly lowered.

The third month – your growing baby

By the end of this month your baby looks just like a little person and is growing rapidly, although his body is still only 5–7 cm (2–3 in) long. The major part of his development is now complete, and the important organs and structures in his body are now formed, although they will carry on developing and growing throughout the rest of the pregnancy. His brain, nervous system and digestive system are all now developing.

Your baby's sex

The sex of your baby is actually determined at the moment of fertilisation, but in the early days of development it is not possible to tell whether the baby is male or female. By the third month, the external genitalia are growing and it begins to be apparent whether your baby is a boy or a girl.

Your baby's movement

The baby is moving around inside your womb by the end of the first trimester, although you won't be able to feel this yourself for a while yet. His arms and legs are now developed and his joints – ankles, knees, wrists, elbows and shoulders – have formed. The fingers and toes, which were fused, have now separated and even the fingernails and toenails are starting to grow. The baby's eyes, ears and the structure of his face are also formed and his profile is developing.

Twins and multiples

If you are expecting twins, they will be growing in just the same way that a single baby would. Multiple pregnancies are monitored more closely in pregnancy, just to be sure that things are progressing well. There are different types of twin pregnancies, depending on whether they are the result of two separate eggs being fertilised (dizygotic or non-identical twins) or one egg dividing into two (monozygotic or identical twins). Non-identical twins each have their own placenta, but sometimes identical twins share a placenta and may even be developing in the same sac inside the womb.

The third month – changes in you

During the third month of pregnancy, you may still be experiencing many of the signs of early pregnancy, such as sickness or tiredness, but these should gradually begin to fade. By the end of this month, you may find that you start to feel better, particularly if you have been feeling very exhausted or nauseous.

You may still experience some digestive problems, such as heartburn, constipation or flatulence, as well as food cravings or aversions. You will have gained some weight due to the changes in your body, such as the growing size of the womb and the fluid inside it as well as the baby and the enlargement of your breasts. If you hadn't been aware of any physical changes to your body in the first couple of months, you are likely to notice them now as your waist thickens and you gain some weight. Most women find that they have an increased appetite unless they have been suffering badly with nausea.

You may find that your hair changes during pregnancy, either becoming thicker or you may lose more than you usually do (see page 61). There may be changes in your skin pigment too (see page 64), and the veins in your legs and in your breasts may become more noticeable (see page 156). Your blood volume will also increase to meet the needs of your changing body.

Headaches

You may experience headaches or migraines during pregnancy, but these will usually ease during the latter half. Feeling tired or stressed can make you more prone to headaches, so it is important to try to get plenty of sleep and to do what you can to help yourself feel more relaxed. Although headaches during pregnancy are quite common as they can be caused by changes in your hormones, you should discuss it with your GP or midwife if you are getting a lot of bad headaches as this can be linked with high blood pressure.

The Second Trimester

The fourth month

This month marks the start of a new phase of your pregnancy as you enter the second trimester. This is a time of change for you and your baby as you gradually begin to look more pregnant and your baby grows steadily.

Feeling more relaxed

You may find that you now start to feel more relaxed and comfortable with your pregnancy at the beginning of the second trimester, and you may feel able to enjoy it much more than up until now. If you have been plagued by sickness, nausea and tiredness, these symptoms often start to fade after the first 12 weeks of pregnancy. There is also a sense of reassurance in the knowledge that the risk of losing the pregnancy is now greatly reduced, as most miscarriages occur during the first 12 weeks.

Researching antenatal classes

Although you may feel that you are still in the fairly early stages of pregnancy, it is a good idea to research antenatal classes at this stage if you plan to take them later on (see page 126). In some areas there is less pressure on places, but in others it may not be easy to find a space if you leave it until late in your pregnancy. It's worth going along to some kind of antenatal class as not only will this be an excellent source of information and advice, it's also a good way to meet other new parents who live nearby. Once you have your baby, it will be invaluable to know others with babies of the same age as yours and this can be a great source of support. Many women and their children make lasting friendships via their antenatal classes.

You may want to investigate other classes that you could attend too, as some are suitable from early in the second trimester. Pregnancy yoga, pregnancy aqua fitness and active birth classes may all be on offer, and it is a good idea to check out what's available in your area and whether the classes might be of interest to you. As with the antenatal classes, going along to a pregnancy fitness or exercise class will not only help you feel better prepared, but may also be a good way to get to know other women who are at the same stage of pregnancy.

The fourth month – your growing baby

Your baby is about the size of your fist by the end of this month, and is somewhere around 20–25 cm (8–10 in) long. The baby's weight can vary quite a bit, but he may weigh up to 226 g (8 oz) by the end of the fourth month.

His arms and legs are longer now, and he even has fingernails. His teeth are starting to develop, too. His skin is a pinky colour and is still very thin and transparent. His head has now moved up and is no longer resting on his chin, and his face is becoming more recognisably 'human' as his features develop.

His genitalia have developed and it may be possible to tell his gender from a scan at this stage of pregnancy. You may or may not decide that you want to know the gender of your baby before the birth – some people like to know, while others prefer a surprise (see also page 157). The placenta has grown and is now producing hormones that are needed during pregnancy. The placenta also helps to protect the baby as it offers a barrier against any infection. The baby's own system is still developing rapidly too – he is even starting to urinate into the amniotic fluid.

Noticeable movements

Your baby is moving around much more now, and as he grows you may start to feel his movements towards the end of this month. It's often hard to identify these movements at first as they are slight and you may not be sure whether it is really the baby moving at all or just a gurgling in your tummy. It may feel like a 'fluttering' sensation, or a bit like bubbles. Gradually, as you feel more movements, you will become more accustomed to them and be able to recognise them. Once you become aware of the movements, don't expect your baby to keep moving around all the time. He will have periods when he is sleeping or resting and other, more active, times. The movements you feel will grow stronger and more easily recognisable with time, as your baby grows bigger. Once you are aware of movements, don't forget to involve your partner in experiencing them (see page 247).

The fourth month – changes in you

By the end of this month, the changes in your body will be more apparent. Your waist will be thickening and your breasts will probably be growing larger, too. You may find it increasingly difficult to squeeze into some of your normal clothes and may already be wearing maternity clothing, especially if you have been pregnant before, as your skin is less elastic second time around and your abdomen will expand more quickly. Many maternity clothes are cleverly designed to be adjustable, so that they grow with you during pregnancy, and so they may be more comfortable – even if you don't feel particularly big just yet. If you don't feel ready for maternity clothes but are having difficulty fitting into your normal things, perhaps buy ordinary clothes in a larger size rather than special maternity wear. This can be practical for after the birth, when you may need slightly larger clothes, as it usually takes a while to get back to your original size. 'Bump bands' are a great way to fill in the gaps that can occur when tops don't meet up with bottom halves during pregnancy.

Symptoms you may experience

Many of the earlier signs of pregnancy may continue during this month, although the sickness and tiredness often start to fade. There are some other symptoms you may experience, including:

- Swelling in your ankles or feet. This happens because you have more fluid in your body than usual, and it's often more pronounced if you have been standing for a long while or if the weather is very hot. You will usually start to feel much better if you can sit with your feet raised for a while, and you may be able to avoid getting swollen feet if you try not to remain standing for long periods of time. Talk to your GP or midwife straight away if you experience sudden swelling as it can be a sign of pre-eclampsia (see page 191). If one leg becomes more swollen and painful, it is important to consult your GP in case you have deep-vein thrombosis.

- Bleeding gums when you clean your teeth. Although it isn't uncommon to have swollen or sore gums, which can bleed during pregnancy, it is important to keep on top of any potential problems by continuing to pay regular visits to your dentist. You are entitled to free dental care, which carries on for a while after pregnancy too. This is important as the changing hormones in pregnancy can make your gums more vulnerable to plaque and gum disease. Make sure that you clean and floss your teeth regularly and try to avoid having sweet, sugary foods and drinks. (For more on dental care, see page 57.)

- You may develop a dark line running down your abdomen from your tummy button, which is called the 'linea nigra' (see page 65), or other changes to your skin such as brown patches or tiny red bumps known as 'vascular spiders'. Skin tags and moles (see page 66) may also appear during pregnancy, or existing ones may change or grow. If you have moles and you notice changes in them during pregnancy, you should mention this to your GP so that they can be checked properly. You may also notice that the palms of your hands become red during pregnancy (see page 68).

- Headaches are common during pregnancy as they can be caused by the hormonal changes in your body. If you are experiencing severe headaches, do talk to your GP or midwife about this as they can be an indication of high blood pressure (see page 191). If you want to take a painkiller, paracetamol is generally considered safe to take during pregnancy, but it is worth checking with your pharmacist, GP or midwife before taking any over-the-counter painkillers as some are not suitable to take during pregnancy and it is sensible to check first (see page 87).

- Varicose veins. Your veins may become more noticeable during pregnancy and they can become very pronounced. If this develops into a real problem, you may want to try wearing support tights and you should make sure you don't remain standing for long periods. Varicose veins usually occur in your legs, but sometimes they are found in the birth canal and this can be very uncomfortable.

- Haemorrhoids or piles. It is very common to suffer from haemorrhoids, or dilated blood vessels in or around the anus, during pregnancy. They can get worse as your pregnancy progresses and if they become very uncomfortable or bleed, you should talk to your GP. (Don't use any medication without checking with a pharmacist, GP or midwife that it is suitable for use during pregnancy.) Haemorrhoids are caused partly by the increased weight of the baby, but suffering from constipation, which is common in pregnancy, can make them worse if you strain when you go to the loo. One of the best ways to try to avoid them is to ensure that you have plenty of fibre and fluid in your diet, which will help you to avoid constipation.

- Increased vaginal discharge. This is quite normal during pregnancy, and it doesn't necessarily indicate that you have an infection. You only need to worry if the discharge causes irritation or itching and smells unpleasant, in which case you should see your GP.

- Changes in your breasts. By the start of the second trimester, your breasts will have usually swollen, as they increase in size and in weight. The nipples may grow bigger and the circular area surrounding them (the areola) may grow and begin to change colour, darkening from a pinkish shade to becoming more brown (see also page 64).

The fifth month

By the end of the fifth month, you may have started to feel your baby move about, although initially you may not be sure that it is really the baby that you are feeling. You will soon learn to recognise your baby's movements.

The anomaly scan

You will probably have a scan at the end of this month, when you are between 18 and 20 weeks pregnant. This scan is often referred to as the 'anomaly scan' because it is used to check for any problems, or 'anomalies'. (See page 113 for more on this scan.)

Boy or girl?

It is sometimes possible to find out the sex of your baby at this scan if he or she is lying in the right position, and the sonographer is able to tell you. However, you need to think hard about whether you really want to know or not. You may also be given, or be allowed to purchase, a photo of the scan image of your baby. If any potential problems are identified during this scan, you will usually be referred to a specialist in foetal medicine.

The fifth month – your growing baby

Your baby will have grown considerably, and by the end of this month he will be approaching 0.5 kg (1 lb) in weight, but he would not yet be able to survive outside your body. He will be moving about a lot by this time, as his nervous system and muscles are now more developed. As he's still quite small there is plenty of room for him to perform gymnastics in your tummy, so you are likely to be aware of his movements. He is able to feel pressure on your tummy and may move in reaction to it.

Your baby doesn't have any fat on his body at first, and layers of fatty tissue begin to build up during this month. This fat is important as it helps him to keep warm and also helps to regulate his temperature, which is essential once he is born.

Vernix caseosa

Your baby's body is covered in a creamy substance called 'vernix caseosa', which is a waxy covering that helps to protect his skin. He needs this as he is floating about in the amniotic fluid and it stops his skin peeling or wrinkling up. The vernix caseosa is produced by the sebaceous glands in his skin and it also has anti-biotic qualities to help to ward off any infection.

Lanugo

The hair is starting to grow on his head and his eyelashes and eyebrows are developing. His body is also covered in a fine, downy layer of hair, which is called 'lanugo'. Babies sometimes start sucking their thumbs at this stage.

Reproductive organs

The baby's sex organs become more developed during this stage of pregnancy. If you are expecting a boy, his testicles will begin to descend and, amazingly, a baby girl will already have several million immature eggs in her ovaries – the most that they will ever hold. By the time she is born, this number will be reduced to about two million and many will continue to perish throughout her life. By the time she reaches puberty there will be about half a million remaining, at most. On average, she will release one of these eggs each month as part of her menstrual cycle, but the majority of the immature eggs in the ovaries will never develop.

Recognising sounds

Parents often claim that their newborns seem to recognise certain music or particular sounds that they have heard when they were still in the womb. From this stage of pregnancy, your baby's hearing is developing and he is able to hear all the noises that your body makes, but also things outside your body too. You could start playing music or singing to your unborn baby, so that special pieces of music or songs are familiar to him once he is born. Some parents have found that this familiar music is very soothing to the baby in the early days, weeks and months after birth.

The fifth month – changes in you

You will put on weight more rapidly from this stage of pregnancy onward, as your baby grows. You no longer have a waistline as your bump becomes rounded and you will be more comfortable wearing maternity clothes.

Stretch marks

You may start to develop stretch marks at this stage of pregnancy as your skin stretches to accommodate your growing baby (see page 64). You may not like the look of them, but stretch marks do not cause any problems and nine out of ten women get them during pregnancy.

There are many products on the market that claim to help prevent stretch marks, but it's the pregnancy hormones in your body that affect your skin and make you more prone to getting stretch marks at this time, so there is not much you can do to prevent them in the first place. Generally, one of the best ways to reduce their effects is to make sure that you gain weight gradually (see page 37). Sometimes women are encouraged to 'eat for two' when they are pregnant and this can lead to excessive weight gain, which it is then hard to shift after the baby is born. Sticking to a good, healthy diet is essential, and this will reduce your chances of getting stretch marks. Massaging your stomach with a good moisturiser is also a good idea as it is soothing for you and helps build a connection between you and your bump, although is unlikely to prevent you getting the marks altogether.

Your diet

When you are pregnant you'll probably find that your appetite increases. In fact, you only need about an extra 200 calories a day (see page 37), so while it can be tempting to assume that this means you can eat more chocolate bars, sweets or 'unhealthy' snacks, it is very important to try to make sure that the extra calories you consume are still part of a healthy, balanced diet with lots of fresh fruit and vegetables (see Chapter 3).

Frequent, small meals

You probably will no longer be feeling sick or nauseous by this stage of your pregnancy, but you may have problems with indigestion, heartburn or reflux. Rather than sticking to three large meals a day, you may find that any digestive problems in pregnancy are helped if you eat smaller meals more frequently. Fatty, spicy or fried foods often make digestive problems worse and you may feel better if you avoid these.

Breathlessness

By this stage, you may find that you are becoming short of breath more quickly after exercise. This is quite common in pregnancy, and doesn't mean that you need to stop exercising altogether, although you may want to take things more gently and slowly. Breathlessness is not usually a problem unless it is very severe and you feel faint after activity, or if you are having palpitations or chest pains or are finding it hard to breathe when you are lying down. If you have any of these symptoms, you should see your GP.

Swollen gums

Having swollen or spongy gums is quite common by this stage of pregnancy and you may find that your gums bleed when you clean your teeth. It is important to visit your dentist at least once while you are pregnant to have a check-up and there should be no charge for this. (See page 58 for more on this.)

Iron deficiency

You may suffer from iron deficiency during pregnancy, which can lead to anaemia (see page 178), making you feel very tired or dizzy. If you are worried about this, try to eat more foods that are rich in iron such as spinach, iron-fortified cereals, beef, blackstrap molasses, prune juice or dried fruit, potatoes, white beans and pumpkin seeds. If your iron levels are low, your GP or midwife may recommend an iron supplement.

The sixth month

You are now in the last stages of the second trimester of pregnancy and you may be starting to get ready for your baby's arrival. You may begin to feel tired and uncomfortable as your belly grows bigger to accommodate your baby. By the end of this month, you are two-thirds of the way through your pregnancy and you will be thinking about the birth as you head towards the home straight.

The sixth month – your growing baby

Your baby will usually weigh about 800 g (1¾ lb) by the end of this month and will be around 35 cm (14 in) long.

Your baby's reflexes are developing and he is able to hiccup. Nerves in his ears are more fully developed, so that he can hear your voice and may even respond to touch and sound from outside the womb. His eyes are beginning to open now. There is not much to see inside your womb, but he may respond to bright light outside your body. He is already developing sleep patterns and you may start to notice that he is more active at certain times of the day. His movements will be growing stronger as he practises stretching and kicking. This may be quite uncomfortable for you at times, especially if he always seems to move just as you are settling down to rest.

Breathing movements

Your baby will be making breathing movements by now, practising inhaling and exhaling – to help develop his lungs. As he does these practice breaths, he takes small quantities of the amniotic fluid in and out, getting ready for real breathing once he is born.

Survival

If your baby happened to be born prematurely at the end of this month, he would have a chance of surviving, although he would need intensive neonatal care because his lungs and some of his other organs would not yet be properly developed.

The sixth month – changes in you

You will be very aware of your bump by now and you may start to feel uncomfortable. It is likely that you experience some aches and pains, your feet and ankles may be prone to swelling and you may have cramps in your legs (see page 76).

Constipation

Many women suffer from constipation at this stage of pregnancy. It's partly due to the fact that your progesterone levels are high and this can slow down your digestion because it relaxes the muscles throughout your body. Constipation can lead to haemorrhoids, which are a common problem during pregnancy (see page 156). Trying to make sure that you eat more fibre, keeping your fluid intake up and taking plenty of exercise will all help reduce the risk of developing constipation.

Heartburn

The relaxed muscles in your digestive system can also cause heartburn and you may find that you start to feel bloated, which you may be able to resolve by eating regular, small meals rather than three large ones each day (see also page 77).

Feeling forgetful

Many women feel that they become forgetful by this stage of pregnancy and you may hear people describe the 'fuzziness' they experience as 'pregnancy brain'. It has been suggested that this absent-mindedness is mainly due to the fact that you are preoccupied with thoughts about your baby, but some women do find it causes difficulties, such as when driving. Getting more sleep may help and if you are feeling forgetful, try to note things down which will jog your memory about important things.

Clumsiness

You may also feel that you are more clumsy than normal, as your increased girth and weight, along with loosened joints, can lead you to trip over or bang into things more easily, which could be dangerous. Taking things generally more slowly may help – remember you are not the same size or shape as you were just a few months ago.

Backache

Backache is also quite common during pregnancy, as your body's joints and ligaments all become more relaxed. If you are experiencing backache, try to be careful about how you move, taking care to bend your knees rather than your back if you need to pick things up. You may also find that you have some aches in your lower abdomen as everything grows and stretches to make space for your baby.

Braxton Hicks contractions

Although your baby's birth is still some months away, you may start experiencing Braxton Hicks contractions by the end of the second trimester. These contractions occur when the muscles in the womb tighten and you may feel your bump becoming suddenly hard and taut. The contractions aren't painful and they usually only last for a minute at most. They are unpredictable and irregular, and actually start occurring just a few weeks into pregnancy, although you won't be able to feel them until your womb has grown larger.

There are a number of theories as to why pregnant women experience Braxton Hicks contractions as part of a preparation for labour. Some believe they help to soften the cervix and others suggest that they help to tone up the muscles in your womb. Women sometimes worry that they won't be able to distinguish real contractions from the Braxton Hicks ones, but real contractions become more frequent and regular, are more painful and last longer. Braxton Hicks contractions can be uncomfortable, but will often cease if you move about.

The Third Trimester

You are now getting ready for the birth of your baby and you can look forward to his arrival. Try not to feel too anxious about the birth, but instead ensure that you make the most of these last weeks of peace and quiet before your new baby arrives.

The final months of pregnancy can drag and you may feel emotional at this point, when it often seems that all you can do is wait for your baby to arrive. It can be particularly difficult if your pregnancy continues past your due date. This can be a frustrating time as you may not be able to do much and all you can focus on is the imminent arrival of your baby. You may start to feel anxious about the birth and about your baby, whether you will bond with him and whether you are capable of being a good mother. These worries and concerns are all very common and real.

Get as much rest as you can and try to enjoy time with your partner, in preparation for the huge changes that lie ahead.

The seventh month

The third trimester marks the last three months of pregnancy and by this stage you will be starting to think ahead to the birth and planning for life with your new baby. By the start of the seventh month you will probably feel fairly large even though your baby will still have quite a lot more growing to do.

The seventh month – your growing baby

At the start of the third trimester, your baby probably weighs about 1 kg (2 lb) and during the seventh month he will grow rapidly, gaining weight as he fills out. Until this point he has possessed very little body fat, but the fat underneath his skin begins to grow at this stage of pregnancy and he will need it to keep him warm once he is born. The fat will also help smooth out his skin so he will be less wrinkly.

Babies born at this stage of pregnancy need a lot of special care, but most survive. Although most of the important structures and organs in their bodies are fully formed by this stage in pregnancy, the lungs are still immature. Premature babies often experience problems with breathing because of this and often need help with it for a while. They are at risk of respiratory problems.

Feeling your baby moving

You will feel your baby moving as he practises kicking and stretching and these movements will be stronger now, but they may be less frequent. He still has some room to move about in the womb, although this will gradually decrease over the next couple of months. He won't necessarily be in the right position for birth yet, with his head downwards. You may feel him hiccupping, which is usually the result of swallowing amniotic fluid.

Eyes and head

His eyes have now developed and he can open and close them. They will react to light, but he won't learn how to focus properly until he is born. His eyebrows are forming at this stage too. His body is still covered in fine, downy hair and he also has more hair growing on his head. Your baby's brain is developing rapidly this month as he begins to be able to taste and to feel pain.

The seventh month – changes in you

By the seventh month of pregnancy, your tummy will be rounded and you may feel increasingly uncomfortable as the ligaments stretch to accommodate your growing baby. Your tummy button may turn inside out as your abdomen fills out. The stretched skin of your stomach may feel itchy and you may find that you start to get backache as the weight of the baby increases.

You may also suffer from some of the problems of digestion such as constipation, indigestion, heartburn and bloating. You may find that you start to feel much more hungry as your baby is growing rapidly and your breasts may feel much fuller now as your body prepares for breast-feeding.

Make a birth plan

Tiredness could be a problem at this point. There still seems to be quite a way to go before the birth and you may be getting impatient and concerned about it. If you haven't already, it's a good idea to start making plans for the birth with a birth plan (see page 128). It is important to remember that once you are in labour, it may not be possible to follow this plan exactly, since giving birth is unpredictable, but it is still a good idea to think through what you would prefer, ideally – if things go as you would like.

Antenatal checks

You will be receiving regular antenatal checks, and your midwife will be monitoring your blood pressure and checking your urine. She will also listen to the baby's heartbeat and establish his position by feeling your abdomen. Don't worry if your baby hasn't settled into his birth position yet, as it is quite common for babies to still be lying across the womb at this stage of pregnancy.

The eighth month

By this stage, you will start to feel as if you are heading towards the home straight. With just weeks to go until your baby arrives, you will probably feel very large and quite tired by this point. You may have already given up work and started your maternity leave (see page 263) or you may be looking forward to this, and it's a good idea to relax as much as you can in preparation for the busy time ahead. You will continue to have regular checks with your midwife to make sure that things are still progressing as they should be.

The eighth month – your growing baby

Your baby is starting to get ready for the birth by the eighth month of pregnancy. His organs are developed by this stage and his bones are getting stronger too. His lungs are not entirely ready to operate fully at this point, and a baby born in the eighth month may still need some help with breathing at first.

Your baby now sleeps properly, going into phases of deep sleep, and you will probably notice times when he is awake and active – perhaps even seeing a regular pattern in his movements. He is a lot bigger now and may weigh as much as 2.25 kg (5 lb). There isn't much room for him to move about inside the womb and so he will start moving less.

This is a time of rapid weight gain and he will continue to grow heavier throughout the next few weeks until the birth, gaining as much as 226 g (8 oz) every week.

The baby is so big by this point that you may feel quite uncomfortable as he presses up against your ribs. Once he moves into position ready for birth, with his head facing downwards, you may find that you feel much more comfortable.

The eighth month – changes in you

Many women find that they are quite tired by the eighth month of pregnancy, but may also find that they don't always sleep well, as it can be hard to find a comfortable position at night (see page 74).

The baby now takes up so much space that you are likely to feel quite breathless and need to urinate frequently if he is pressing against your bladder. It can feel more comfortable once he moves down into position ready for the birth. This new position, along with the fact that your joints are all more flexible and relaxed, can affect the way that you walk and you may feel that you have started to 'waddle'. Walking, or waddling, can feel quite uncomfortable by this stage, but it is important to try to keep taking some gentle exercise. You may enjoy swimming now as the water makes you feel weightless (see page 98), and yoga classes for pregnancy are a popular form of exercise in the final months of pregnancy (see page 97).

Colostrum

As your body gets ready to feed your baby, you may notice a discharge of yellow fluid, called 'colostrum', from your nipples. This doesn't happen to everyone, but it is quite common during the third trimester. Colostrum is a nutritious liquid, which is the ideal food for your baby during his first few days of life, helping to protect him from infection. If you find that leaking is a problem, you may want to buy some special nursing pads (see page 228).

Braxton Hicks

If you haven't noticed them already, you may become aware of Braxton Hicks contractions where your body gets ready for the birth (see page 165). You can experience these as a tightening of your bump and they may be uncomfortable. They are not the same as the contractions you feel in labour, as they are not usually painful and are irregular.

The ninth month

You are now in the final few weeks of pregnancy and will be looking forward to your due date eagerly, but perhaps accompanied with some anxiety too. Remember that most babies aren't born precisely on their due date, which is more a guide than an exact timing, and it is normal for babies to arrive two weeks on either side of that date (see also page 28). You will probably have weekly appointments with your midwife during this final stage of pregnancy, and may find that you are increasingly keen for your baby to arrive, as you feel heavier and more uncomfortable. It is common to feel that you just want to move on to the next stage.

Your midwife will probably advise you to keep your hospital bag packed (see overleaf) and ready, with all that you need for the birth during this last month, so that you are prepared for your baby's arrival.

The ninth month – your growing baby

Your baby is still growing bigger and gaining weight during the ninth month. The average baby weighs around 3.4 kg (7½ lb) at birth, but it is perfectly normal for a baby to weigh more or less than this.

Your baby has very little space to move around inside the womb now, and he has to curl up quite tightly to fit. He may drop further down so that his head lies very low in your pelvis, ready for the birth.

Meconium

Your baby's body will start to produce meconium in these last few weeks. This is a sticky black or dark-green substance, which is what he has ingested while inside you. His first bowel movement after birth will consist of meconium, although this can sometimes happen during the birth itself.

Your hospital bag

Use this checklist to make sure that you have everything you need when you go into hospital. Gathering everything together in advance will prevent you having a last-minute panic.

- Books, magazines, music
- Snacks such as cereal bars, nuts, fruit
- Drinks (boxed drinks with straws)
- Lip salve
- Massage oil
- TENS machine (if desired)
- Your maternity notes
- Your birth plan
- Cotton nightdresses that undo down the front
- Lightweight dressing gown
- Socks
- Slippers
- Watch
- Water spray
- Face cloth
- Hairband or clips
- Pillow
- Towel, hairbrush
- Earplugs
- Camera
- Phone
- Toiletries and wash bag
- Inflatable birthing ball (if desired)
- Nursing bras and breast pads
- Maternity sanitary pads
- Underwear
- Comfortable clothes for your return home
- Nappies
- Cotton Wool
- Baby clothes
- Baby hat, socks, jacket
- Shawl
- Muslin squares
- Small amount of cash and loose change
- Baby car seat

Organs and hair

His organs are now all fully developed and even his lungs are ready to breathe. The hair that has covered his entire body will gradually be shed during this month. He is now just waiting to be born.

The ninth month – changes in you

The last few weeks of pregnancy can be tough for a mother-to-be. You will feel large and often uncomfortable and may find that you are suffering from all kinds of pregnancy-related aches and pains, from backache to pressure in your pelvis. You may find it hard to sleep as it is often difficult to get into a comfortable position (see page 74) and also you may need to keep getting up to go to the loo.

The weight of the baby at the front of your body can make you feel ungainly as your centre of gravity has now shifted. You may find yourself leaning backwards to try to compensate for the extra weight at the front of your body and this can make you feel unbalanced and clumsy.

The skin on your tummy is stretched very tightly now and it may feel itchy and uncomfortable. You may notice a vaginal discharge as the plug of mucus from the cervix thins out and the cervix itself softens ready for birth.

You may suffer from indigestion in the last month of pregnancy and find that eating smaller, more frequent, meals is easier for your body (see also page 77).

Nesting instinct

It is quite common for women to be struck by a 'nesting instinct' just before they go into labour. If you find yourself unexpectedly needing to start clearing out the kitchen cupboards or loft, this may well be a sign that your baby will arrive before too long. Try not to overdo things as you don't want to be exhausted when the time comes to give birth.

Your emotions in the last weeks

The last few weeks of pregnancy can be a strange time emotionally. You may find that you start to feel very impatient, particularly if your due date comes and goes without any sign of your baby arriving, and you may be longing for the birth so that you can get on with your new life. You may feel very large and exhausted and this can make the last few weeks quite difficult as it takes more time to get normal things done.

You may be feeling a little concerned about the birth and how you will cope, or about whether you will bond with your baby and be able to look after him properly. This is only natural, but do try not to get too anxious, since staying calm in the early stages of labour, if possible, will be beneficial.

However, some women find that they feel very contented towards the end of their pregnancy. You cannot rush about too much and you may find that you feel quite relaxed and dreamy. Try to enjoy these last days of peace as much as you can and make the most of them – indulge yourself by resting frequently, as you will need to preserve your energies for the labour and the early days with your new baby.

10

Complications and Problems in Pregnancy

Most pregnancies progress perfectly well without any serious problems, but there are sometimes issues that can crop up. Usually these are fairly minor difficulties that may be quite common during pregnancy but which may need looking at to make sure that everything progresses as it should. Occasionally, there are more complex problems with either yourself or your baby that may need some additional help.

You may find that you get very worried about pregnancy-related problems for both yourself and your baby, and while it is a good idea to be aware of the types of difficulties that can arise, it is important to keep these in perspective and to try not to be too anxious about things. If you are at all worried about anything, consult your GP or your midwife, who will put your mind at rest or arrange treatment for you.

If you suffer from a pre-existing medical condition, it is important that your GP is aware of your full medical history and that it is recorded at your booking visit (see page 106). This is to make sure that you see the appropriate specialist.

Potential difficulties

During pregnancy, your body goes through many dramatic changes and sometimes the extra pressure it is put under can lead to some common complaints. Most of these are not serious, although you may need to take some supplements or some extra care, but sometimes more complicated issues can arise and it is a good idea to be aware of the signs that a problem could be developing.

If you do have any worries or concerns, it is always a good idea to talk to your GP or midwife. Quite often, there will be nothing to worry about. If there is a problem that needs tackling, they will be able to spot what it is, offer to help you and give you the advice you need. Try to keep in mind that, while it would be unusual to go through pregnancy without any kind of discomfort or any minor niggles, serious complications are rare.

Anaemia

Anaemia is all too common in pregnancy and is due to a fall in the number of red blood cells, partly because of the fact that your blood volume increases and dilutes the red blood cells. Anaemia in pregnancy is defined when the haemoglobin level drops below 11 g/dl.

Iron-deficiency anaemia is the most common kind of anaemia in pregnancy, as your growing baby takes much of the iron he needs from you. Anaemia can also occur with folate deficiency, certain hereditary blood disorders, such as thalassaemia, and sickle cell disease and chronic illnesses.

If you are anaemic you may notice that you feel more tired than usual and look a little pale. If you have been eating a good basic healthy diet, you probably won't need to worry. You will be more at risk of anaemia if you are eating a poor diet and/or you have had multiple pregnancies. If you are at risk of anaemia or are anaemic you will be advised to take iron supplements by your GP or midwife. The daily recommended amount is 3 mg. You will also be advised to eat iron-rich foods such as red meat, spinach, fish and chicken.

If your blood count does not improve or if you cannot take oral iron, you may be able to have iron injections and, rarely, intravenous iron or a blood transfusion.

Anxiety and depression

You may find that you experience mood swings in pregnancy. These are not uncommon, often due to the hormonal changes taking place in your body. If you start feeling down for most of the time or find yourself crying a lot, it is worth talking to your GP or midwife. They can offer you counselling and even treatment to help you feel better and cope with your pregnancy. After you have had your baby, you will then be followed up to make sure you do not need treatment for postnatal depression.

Miscarriage

Miscarriage is the death of the foetus before the twenty-fourth week of pregnancy. Losing a pregnancy, even in the very early stages, is distressing and it is quite normal to feel very upset. Sometimes your emotions can be overwhelming, but it is helpful to try to remember that most women who have had a miscarriage do go on to have a healthy and successful pregnancy.

About one in four pregnancies end in miscarriage, but some miscarriages happen so early in the pregnancy that you may not even realise you are pregnant. Your risk of miscarriage increases with age and is as high as 50 per cent for women who are over the age of 40.

Women are often worried about the risk of losing their baby during the first trimester, but it is not unusual to experience some vaginal bleeding or abdominal pain during pregnancy, and this doesn't necessarily mean that you are going to have a miscarriage. However, it is important to see your GP or midwife just to make sure that everything is all right because these can be warning signs.

Many hospitals have early pregnancy units, which you can attend independently or you can be referred to one by your GP. If there are any concerns, you will be usually be offered an ultrasound scan as this can give a reliable assessment as to whether there is a problem.

If the scan indicates that the pregnancy has been lost, this is known as a 'complete' miscarriage, and no treatment will be necessary. If you are told that you have had an 'incomplete' miscarriage this means that some pregnancy tissue remains and you may need additional medical care.

There are several options for treatment. A surgical procedure called evacuation of retained products (ERPC) may be recommended after an incomplete miscarriage, especially if there was continued bleeding. This procedure is usually done under a general anaesthetic and involves passing a fine suction tube into the uterus and removing the remaining tissue.

If you are not bleeding heavily and there are no signs of infection, you may be given the option of waiting to see if you have a complete miscarriage, so that you can avoid having surgery. Alternatively, you may be offered a vaginal or oral tablet of a drug called Misoprostol. If you take this, you will be able to go home and just come back for follow-up scans to ensure that no remaining tissue is left. Sometimes if you choose to wait or take Misoprostol, there is still a risk that it may be necessary to carry out an ERPC later if there is some remaining tissue.

Ectopic pregnancy

In some pregnancies the fertilised egg will become implanted in the tube rather than in your womb. This is known as an 'ectopic' pregnancy. If this happens, the pregnancy will never be able to develop as it is not possible for an embryo to grow in the tube, but it can be risky for you as there is a danger that the pregnancy can rupture the tube.

If you experience abdominal pain, particularly on one side more than the other, or vaginal bleeding, you should contact your GP or hospital to be seen as soon as possible. Sometimes the bleeding may look unusual and some women describe it as being 'dark' or 'watery like prune juice'.

You may be at increased risk of an ectopic pregnancy if you have had:

- In vitro fertilisation (IVF) treatment.

- A previous history of pelvic infection/major abdominal surgery.

- The intrauterine contraceptive device (IUCD)/are taking the mini-pill.

- A previous history of surgery to your tubes.

- A previous ectopic pregnancy.

If you have pain and bleeding in early pregnancy, you will need to have an ultrasound scan. If the scan shows that the foetus is growing well in the uterus, there will be no reason for further concern, but if the pregnancy is ectopic you will be offered treatment. Sometimes it is difficult to know whether you have an ectopic pregnancy in the early days, and a repeat scan and blood test may be necessary to be quite sure.

If your ectopic pregnancy is not far advanced and there is no obvious bleeding you may be offered a drug called Methotrexate, which will reduce risk of bleeding and rupture of your tube. If this is not an option, surgery may be necessary. You will need a general anaesthetic and the operation will usually be carried out using a keyhole surgery technique known as a laparoscopy; small cuts are made in the abdomen and the surgeon carries out the operation using instruments through these cuts attached to a camera. Sometimes it is possible to remove the ectopic pregnancy without removing the tube, but otherwise it may be necessary to remove it entirely. Occasionally, if the operation cannot be done by laparoscopy, a small cut low in your abdomen may be needed. Even if one of the tubes is removed, it is still possible for you to get pregnant naturally in the future as long as the other hasn't been damaged or removed.

After an ectopic pregnancy, it is normal to feel worried about the chance of a future pregnancy. Remember that most women who experience an ectopic pregnancy go on to have normal healthy pregnancies.

Backache and musculo-skeletal problems

Backache and muscular pains are very common in pregnancy as your ligaments soften in order to support your baby. Your girth and weight increase and there is a shift in your centre of gravity as you progress in pregnancy. It is important that you are careful when you lift heavy objects, bending from your knees, to make sure that you do not strain your back even more. Sitting straight rather than hunched, avoiding crossing your knees, wearing flat shoes and maintaining a good posture all help.

You may notice more pain when you walk or move your hips. This happens because of a separation of the pubic bones and the hip joints (symphysis pubis diastasis). If this is severe and affecting your ability to move around then see your GP, who will refer you to a physiotherapist. They can give you helpful aids for reducing the discomfort, such as walking aids and a support belt. This condition usually rights itself again once your baby is born and it should not affect you having a normal delivery.

Carpal tunnel syndrome
Carpal tunnel syndrome occurs when the median nerve running from the forearm to your wrist gets compressed in the tight space of the carpal tunnel near the wrist. This makes your hand weak and you may experience a tingling sensation. A splint may help relieve this discomfort so consult your GP.

Bleeding
If you experience bleeding late on in your pregnancy you should always see your GP urgently. Although the risk of miscarriage is less common after 12 weeks have gone by, there are other reasons why bleeding can occur, such as if the placenta is low.

Placenta praevia
This is more common if you have had a previous Caesarean section. It is when the placenta is positioned low in the uterus and is very near, or actually covering, your cervix. If the placenta

is low, you will be advised to have a repeat scan to make sure that it has moved up the womb. For most women this does happen. If by the later stages of pregnancy the placenta is very near your cervix or actually covering it, you will probably be advised to have a Caesarean section. It is safer to avoid having sex at this stage. Be careful about going on long journeys if you are going to be a distance away from a hospital – if you start bleeding you will need to be seen urgently.

Placental abruption

This is not common and occurs when the placenta separates from the uterus. You will experience abdominal pain, your uterus will be tender and tense and you may feel very unwell. You may not have any bleeding. If you experience anything similar to this, contact your GP without delay as your baby may have to be delivered straight away.

Pre-term labour

Sometimes bleeding can occur if your cervix opens in early labour. If this is happens, accompanied by a thick mucous discharge and you are near your due date, it is called a 'show' (see page 281). If it is earlier in the pregnancy and you have contraction-like pains it may be that you are in pre-term labour and you should go to hospital to be examined urgently.

If you experience bleeding, especially if it is accompanied by pain, you should see your GP. You will be assessed in hospital and your baby will be monitored. Most cases of bleeding usually settle without any intervention being necessary. If you are rhesus-negative an injection of anti-D will be given (see page 206).

Infections

There are a number of infections that can occur in pregnancy and some of these may be riskier than if you were not pregnant because your natural immunity is reduced. Some infections may affect your baby, as described below.

Flu
Whatever stage of pregnancy you have reached, you should be offered the seasonal flu vaccine. This is because as a pregnant woman you are more prone to complications from flu, which can cause very serious illness for both you and your baby, such as severe breathing difficulties and pneumonia. You are at particular risk if you have a pre-existing chest problem such as asthma or are on immunosuppressant drugs.

Chickenpox
Most women are immune to chickenpox, but if you are not sure whether you are or not it is routinely tested for at your first antenatal visit. It is important that you avoid catching it as chickenpox in pregnancy is much more severe than otherwise. There is a small chance that your baby could be affected with a condition called foetal varicella syndrome. If you are not immune and you come into contact with the infection during pregnancy, you should stay away from other pregnant women until your spots have crusted over. A blood test will confirm whether you have

been infected or not. You will be given an injection of immunoglobulin, which contains antibodies to the chickenpox virus. This may prevent chickenpox from developing, or it produces a much less serious infection if it does develop. It is best to have this within four days of contact with an infected person, but it will work for up to 10 days.

The baby has a risk of foetal varicella syndrome if you catch chickenpox up to 20 weeks in your pregnancy. You will be offered a detailed ultrasound scan at 16–20 weeks of your pregnancy, or five weeks after the infection has cleared, if the infection was later on in your pregnancy, to look for foetal varicella syndrome. If you develop chickenpox within seven days before or after the birth of your baby, there is the risk he can get severe pneumonia if he is infected and so he will be given immunoglobulin treatment.

Shingles occurs as a result of secondary infection and causes lesions on the skin, but these are less infectious. If you are in contact with shingles, the risk of problems in your baby is far reduced.

Whooping cough (Pertussis)

Whooping cough is an infectious respiratory disease that causes severe coughing in adults and can lead to severe respiratory problems and pneumonia in young babies. There is a vaccine for babies at two months but young babies are very susceptible to infection before this time. It is now recommended that all pregnant women should be vaccinated against whooping cough from 28 weeks of pregnancy. To protect your baby, the best time to get vaccinated is between 28 and 38 weeks of pregnancy.

Genital herpes

Genital herpes is caused by a sexually transmitted virus, herpes simplex virus type II (HSV II). It produces painful ulcers around the vagina and vulva and flu-like symptoms. If you have active genital herpes for the first time within six weeks of your expected date there is a chance your baby can become infected and be unwell. You will be offered a Caesarean section (see page 306) to reduce the risk of your baby coming into contact with the herpes during vaginal delivery as the risk of this is high. If you have had herpes in the past and have a recurrent infection in pregnancy, there is much less chance of your baby being infected and this does not usually affect how he will be born. A Caesarean section will not be routinely offered.

Chlamydia

Chlamydia infection is increasing in young women and can result in pelvic inflammation and damage to the fallopian tubes, resulting in infertility. If you are pregnant and have an untreated infection or a new infection with chlamydia you may notice vaginal discharge and lower abdominal pain. Chlamydia in pregnancy can lead to infection in your baby, with problems such as pneumonia, conjunctivitis and ear infections. Antibiotics reduce this risk and while you are being treated your partner should be screened and treated.

Gonorrhoea

This sexually transmitted infection may not give you any symptoms during pregnancy, but it can result in much more severe infection, leading to foetal infection, causing premature birth, conjunctivitis and blindness. Like other sexually transmitted infections, it is essential that a full sexual screen is done on yourself and your partner, who must be treated as well. As co-infection with HIV is more common, HIV testing should be done too.

Rubella

Rubella, or German measles, can have serious consequences in pregnancy and therefore it's vital that all women who intend to get pregnant are checked for their immunity before becoming pregnant. If you are not pregnant and found not to be immune, you will be offered a vaccination. If you get rubella infection in the first three months of pregnancy, this may result in a whole range of birth defects of the brain, heart, ears and eyes.

Cytomegalovirus

This is a common virus infection that is spread through the saliva and urine and may result in very few and non-specific symptoms such as a sore throat and fever. If you become infected with CMV in pregnancy there is a 40 per cent chance that you might pass this to your baby. About 10 per cent of infected babies develop long-term learning difficulties and hearing loss as a result, which may not be evident until some time after birth. If there is a chance you may have been infected with CMV, an amniocentesis (see page 115) can check to see whether your baby has been infected.

Toxoplasmosis

Toxoplasmosis is a rare infection caused by a parasite that can be caught by contact with cat litter, eating raw, cured or undercooked meat or having unpasteurised goat's milk or cheese. If you have a cat already then you may well be immune, otherwise it is advisable to avoid contact with cat litter (or at least always wear rubber gloves when you are handling it or ask someone else to do the job) and the above foods. Symptoms include flu-like symptoms, enlarged lymph nodes, muscle aches and headaches. There is a small chance that your baby can become infected, but the risk lessens the further on in pregnancy you are. Babies infected with toxoplasma may not develop problems for some time and these include learning difficulties and disabilities connected with hearing and sight. If you are concerned that you may have been infected, a blood test can check for immunity and you will be given antibiotics to reduce the risk of your baby becoming infected.

Parvovirus

This viral infection is very common in small children and is often called 'slapped cheek syndrome' due to red cheeks appearing as one of the symptoms. If you catch it in pregnancy there is an increased risk of miscarriage and anaemia in your baby. It can result in excessive fluid around the baby called foetal hydrops.

Parvovirus can result in red cheeks, joint pains and a fine rash. If you are concerned that you have caught this, a blood test can check whether you are already immune. If not, there is only a small chance that your baby will be affected and this risk decreases after 20 weeks of pregnancy.

Group B streptococcus

This is a bacteria that is commonly found in the intestine and vagina and it usually causes no problems. However, if your baby becomes infected he may become very unwell and develop complications such as pneumonia and meningitis.

Group B streptococcus is not routinely screened for in pregnancy as results can fluctuate and even a negative test early in pregnancy does not guarantee that you will not get the bacteria later on.

If you have had a previously affected baby, are known to have Group B streptococcus already or have risk factors for Group B streptococcus (your waters have broken before 37 weeks, have been broken for over 24 hours or you develop infection in labour) you will be offered antibiotics in labour to decrease the chance of your baby being infected. Your baby will be monitored after he is born.

HIV

All pregnant women are offered HIV testing because if you are positive then there are a number of things that can be done to significantly reduce the chance of your baby being infected. If your viral count is low and you are in good health, HIV is unlikely to affect either you or your baby or be an indication to avoid having your baby vaginally. An HIV specialist should be involved in your care to give advice on antiretroviral drugs in pregnancy, how to deliver and postnatal care such as avoiding breast-feeding.

Urinary tract infections

Urinary tract infections are very common in pregnancy and your urine will be checked at each of your antenatal visits for infection, as this is linked to pre-term labour and untreated infection may lead to kidney infection. If you notice that your urine smells or that it hurts to pass urine you must tell your GP and you can be given a course of antibiotics.

Urinary incontinence

The pressure of your pregnant uterus and the effect of pro-gesterone leads to weakness of your pelvic floor, resulting in the common symptoms of stress incontinence – leaking urine when you laugh, cough or exert yourself. It is important that you do regular antenatal pelvic floor exercises (see page 93) to reduce the risk of persistent stress incontinence after you have had your baby.

High blood pressure and pre-eclampsia

At each antenatal visit your blood pressure is checked to ensure that it does not become too high (hypertension) or that there are any signs of pre-eclampsia (hypertension with protein in the urine). First-time mothers, mothers over the age of 40, twin pregnancies, those with diabetes, or those with a previous history of blood pressure are at higher risk of this.

High blood pressure in pregnancy is defined as a blood pressure of >140/90 mmHg on two readings more than four hours apart. If you are diagnosed with hypertension before 20 weeks of pregnancy this is called chronic hypertension and this is seen in between 1 and 5 per cent of pregnancies. It is important to diagnose as this is a risk factor for pre-eclampsia. Hypertension after this time, without protein in the urine, is called gestational hypertension and affects between 3 and 10 per cent of pregnancies.

A number of women with hypertension may develop pre-eclampsia. Mild pre-eclampsia affects up to 10 per cent of pregnancies, with 1–2 per cent being severe.

If you have hypertension then you will be monitored more closely, usually as an outpatient. One of the difficulties with high blood pressure in pregnancy is that you can feel perfectly well without realising that your blood pressure is high.

Pre-eclampsia can affect other systems in the body such as the kidney and liver. It can result in symptoms such as headaches, blurred vision, abdominal pain and swelling of the legs. Your baby's growth may also be affected. Rare risks of pre-eclampsia include eclampsia (fits) and placental abruption (placental bleeding). Both are medical emergencies. If your liver is affected a rare condition called HELLPS syndrome may develop (haemolysis, elevated liver enzymes, low platelet count) and delivery should follow. Therefore pre-eclampsia is taken very seriously as it can be life-threatening if it is left untreated.

The treatment for pre-eclampsia is control of blood pressure and delivery of your baby. In order to time this best you will be carefully monitored. Standard investigations include:

- Urine testing for protein by urine dip-stick testing or measurement of the protein creatinine ratio.

● Kidney and liver function tests.

● Full blood count and clotting tests.

Ultrasound scans are often done to ensure that your baby's growth and blood supply is not affected.

Treatment is delivery of your baby, but oral blood pressure medications may be given first. If your labour/delivery is before 36 weeks, steroid injections may be given to you to help mature the baby's lungs. Delivery is by Caesarean section or induction of labour, whichever is more suitable for you and dependant on the severity of the pre-eclampsia and how many weeks the pregnancy is.

If you have severe pre-eclampsia or eclampsia you will be given an intravenous drug called magnesium sulphate and an intravenous blood-pressure drug. You will be monitored for at least 24–48 hours after delivery because even then your blood pressure can rise.

Diabetes

In pregnancy your levels of blood glucose increase and your body finds it more difficult to cope with sugar. This is because your baby's placenta produces a hormone called human placental lactogen, which acts against insulin. If you already suffer from diabetes you may find that your GP will change the dose of your insulin. Some women become diabetic in pregnancy (have gestational diabetes) and there are some women who are not obviously diabetic but cannot manage their carbohydrate intake in the same way as before.

Risk factors for diabetes include a maternal age of more than 37 years, being of Asian or Afro-Caribbean origin, having a high pre-pregnancy weight, a family history of diabetes, previous diabetes, stillbirth or a history of polycystic ovarian disease.

If you suffered from diabetes before your pregnancy you will be referred to a diabetic team and monitored closely. There is a higher risk of miscarriage, stillbirth and foetal abnormalities plus excessive foetal growth. For you there is an increased risk of pre-eclampsia and effects on kidney function. Making sure that your blood sugar is as well controlled as possible before you become pregnant reduces the risks in pregnancy. Consult your GP or midwife about this.

During pregnancy you will be given blood tests for kidney function and diabetic control. Your baby will be monitored to make sure that he is growing at a normal rate and that there is no excessive fluid surrounding him. You need to be careful about your diet to avoid your sugar going too low or too high and you will be asked to test your blood glucose before and after meals. Usually delivery is timed for around 38 weeks.

If you develop diabetes in pregnancy you will be monitored in much the same way. If your diabetes is stable and managed just with your diet, your pregnancy can continue as normal. However, if you need insulin or are on any of the oral diabetic drugs, you will be offered an induction earlier on, depending on the results of blood tests and scans.

Post-delivery, pregnancy-induced diabetes settles down and all drugs are stopped, however there is an increased lifetime risk of diabetes and formal glucose tests should be arranged by your GP.

Deep-vein thrombosis

In pregnancy there are changes in the blood cells that make them more likely to clot. This is of benefit after delivery as it reduces your risk of heavy bleeding, but the disadvantage of these changes is that you are at increased risk of developing clots in the legs (deep-vein thrombosis), which can occasionally go to the lung (pulmonary embolism).

If you suffer from a pain and/or swelling in your calf or any shortness of breath you should see your GP urgently to be checked for this, since if there is a clot in your lung this can be very dangerous for you. You are at increased risk if you are overweight, smoke, have recently travelled long haul, or if you have a history of clotting problems.

Epilepsy

If you suffer from epilepsy you should try to see your specialist before you become pregnant, so that your medication can be altered to one that is least risky to the baby. It is also advisable that you take an increased dose of 5 mg folic acid (see page 18) per day to reduce the risk of spina bifida in your baby.

Your seizures may actually increase in pregnancy, related to a change in drug levels, and so your neurologist should see you regularly. As some drugs may affect the ability of your blood to clot after delivery, you should be given vitamin K at 36 weeks.

Asthma

If your asthma is well controlled and you are taking your medication, it is unlikely that it will have any effect on your pregnancy. However, if you suffer from severe asthma, there is a small risk of poor growth in your baby, pre-term delivery and pre-eclampsia (see page 191). It is important that you continue to take your medication and, if needed, steroids are safe to use.

Heart problems

During pregnancy your blood volume and heart rate increase and this can result in the development of heart problems or worsen any pre-existing heart condition you may have. Abnormalities of heart rate are common and usually transient and often an adaptation to pregnancy. They rarely result in symptoms or need treatment.

If you had major corrective heart surgery as a child, there is a risk of certain heart rate irregularities with some corrected heart conditions. If you or your partner has had a heart defect, your baby will be offered a detailed heart scan to ensure that the heart is developing normally.

If you have replacement heart valves, you need regular check-ups to ensure that the valves are working well and, if you are taking a blood-thinning agent with metal valves, your blood clotting function will need to be checked.

If you have pre-existing heart disease or have developed heart problems in pregnancy you will need a detailed cardiac scan and a review by a cardiologist to decide what treatment is needed and the safest way to deliver your baby.

Kidney problems

Pregnancy can have an effect on kidney function and if you have a pre-existing kidney disease it is important to discuss this with your GP before getting pregnant. The effect on pregnancy depends on the level of kidney impairment, type of kidney disease, if you have high blood pressure and protein in the urine.

If your kidney function is poor this will increase the risk of you needing dialysis and a transplant as well as increased risk of complications in pregnancy for you and your baby.

If you have had a renal transplant there is an increased risk of infection, high blood pressure, pre-term delivery and poor growth in the baby. If your kidney function is good, the overall outcome for your pregnancy is good, but it needs to be carefully managed with the renal physician as some of the drugs may not be safe to use in pregnancy and need to be changed.

Hepatitis

This is caused by a virus and results in jaundice and effects on the liver enzymes. Hepatitis A is caught by contact with faeces and hepatitis B and C via blood or sexual contact. Hepatitis A does not cause long-term liver problems, but B and C may result in liver damage. These diseases may also lead to infection in your baby and increase the risk of stillbirth and premature birth. If you have these infections, your baby will be vaccinated after he has been delivered. It is also important that your medical team is aware so that they can avoid giving you procedures, such as foetal blood sampling, in labour that may increase the risk of transmission to your baby.

Thyroid problems

This affects one per cent of pregnancies. The thyroid gland becomes larger in pregnancy and can be overactive (hyperthyroid) or underactive (hypothyroid). However, if it is treated, there shouldn't be any consequence for your pregnancy. If you have hypothyroidism you will be given thyroid supplements and only if you are undertreated can this lead to foetal problems. If you suffer from hyperthyroidism, you will be given antithyroid drugs, but these can cross the placenta and lead to enlargement of the baby's thyroid (goitre), making him become hypothyroid. The baby should have regular ultrasound scans and his thyroid gland and thyroid function checked to exclude this.

As the level of thyroid hormones can change in pregnancy, your thyroid hormones will be checked throughout your pregnancy and after your baby's delivery to make sure that your drug doses do not need to be altered.

Blood disorders

There are a number of disorders of the blood that happen in pregnancy that lead to alterations in the structure and function of the haemoglobin molecule. The two most common forms are sickle cell disease and thalassaemia and all pregnant women are screened for these.

Sickle cell disease is an inherited disorder of the red blood cells common in people from sub-Saharan Africa and the Middle East. The sickle gene results in abnormal haemoglobin formation. The severe form of the disease is sickle cell disease, where you have both the genes for haemoglobin and the abnormal sickle cell gene. Sickle cell trait is more common and occurs when only one abnormal sickle cell gene is carried. This does not usually affect pregnancy. Sickle cell disease is often diagnosed in childhood and is associated with anaemia, chest problems, infections, stroke and joint pains. If you suffer from any of these conditions, your pregnancy may be high risk and need to be managed in conjunction with a haematologist. Symptoms often get worse in pregnancy and there is an increased risk of pre-eclampsia and thrombosis.

Ideally if you suffer from sickle cell disease you should be seen by your GP before you become pregnant so that your drugs can be reviewed. Prophylactic antibiotics are recommended to reduce the risk of infection. To reduce the risk of folate deficiency you should take 5 mg per day. Aspirin is advised to reduce the risk of pre-eclampsia and you should take the influenza vaccine.

It is possible to screen your partner for the sickle cell gene to determine the risk to your baby. If your partner carries the gene, then diagnostic tests can be done earlier on the baby to see if he is affected. Risks to the baby include poor growth and premature delivery.

The thalassaemias are a group of blood disorders where the production of functional haemoglobin is impaired. There are several different types and these are more common in Asian and Mediterranean people. Thalassaemia may give you a few problems, such as anaemia, but in its most severe form it can affect your baby and result in severe anaemia and excessive fluid accumulation, known as hydrops fetalis. Just like sickle cell disease, you and your partner can be screened and if necessary your baby can be given prenatal testing.

Foetal problems in pregnancy

Although you may want to be aware of the problems that can arise for your baby during pregnancy, it is important to keep these in perspective. When you are pregnant, it is common to worry about whether your baby is all right, but remember that most complications are very rare, and the majority of babies are born without problems.

Pre-term labour and pre-term rupture of membranes

Pre-term labour is when labour happens before 37 weeks. There are a number of risk factors for this such as previous pre-term delivery or late miscarriage, multiple pregnancy, previous surgery on the cervix, previous late terminations of pregnancy, use of recreational drugs, collagen diseases, autoimmune diseases and recurrent urinary tract infections. However, it can occur sporadically when there are no obvious risk factors for pre-term delivery.

The symptoms you may notice are the onset of painful contractions. Pre-term labour may occur with the waters around the baby breaking (pre-term rupture of membranes). If you notice these symptoms you need to contact your hospital to be assessed. You will be examined and an internal examination will be done to check whether the cervix is dilating and to see if the waters have broken. You may notice a watery vaginal discharge. A swab will be taken for a marker called fibronectin. This is produced by the foetal membranes and if this is positive you are at higher risk of actually progressing in labour. If it is negative you have a reduced risk.

You may well not be in labour and you may simply be observed. However, if you are then a drug will be given to help stop the labour. If you are under 36 weeks two steroid injections will be given to help mature the baby's lungs, if you are going to deliver him soon.

If your waters have broken you will be observed for infection with a temperature chart and blood tests. If there is a sign of infection, you may be advised that it is best to deliver your baby now. It is thought that infection is the underlying cause for many cases of pre-term labour and ruptured membranes. In general, if your blood tests and temperature are fine you will be monitored with twice-weekly blood tests as an outpatient and you will be shown how to monitor your temperature and look for signs of infection. Antibiotics are recommended as there is evidence that they reduce the risks to both you and your baby. Most hospitals recommend that if you have not delivered by 34 weeks, then your delivery should be planned for soon after this time. If possible the best way for this is for your labour to be induced and to aim for a vaginal delivery.

It is important that if there is a high chance that the baby will be delivered at less than 37 weeks that you deliver in a unit which has the expertise to look after the baby. You may need to be transferred and give birth in a unit that has the space and specialised staff to look after the baby. The level of paediatric expertise needed is higher the younger the baby is. Usually there is nothing to worry about and survival rates are very good, but babies who are delivered at less than 28 weeks may need special care as their lungs and major organs are not fully mature.

If you have had a pre-term delivery or late miscarriage before, a cervical length scan can be done early in pregnancy. A shorter cervical length is related to a high risk of pre-term delivery. You may be offered a cervical stitch.

Small babies

A baby can be small if his growth has slowed down or stopped (intrauterine growth restriction) or he can be constitutionally small ('small mum, small baby'). At each antenatal visit the height of your uterus will be measured to see if there is a discrepancy between the size of the uterus and your dates. An ultrasound will be done if there is a discrepancy. If you are small yourself you may well have a smaller-than-average baby and this is normal and healthy for you.

Your baby may be more predisposed to growth problems if you have a chronic disease, are an older mum, have a multiple pregnancy, smoke, have raised blood pressure, have certain blood disorders or use alcohol and drugs. In the baby, risk factors include chromosomal abnormalities, intra-uterine infection and poor placental function.

If it is suspected that your baby is small an ultrasound will be done to measure his growth, estimate his weight and assess the fluid around him and the blood flow to the placenta. The ultrasound scans plot the baby's growth on centile charts that are population charts giving average weights of babies at different gestations. Therefore 10 per cent of babies are under the tenth centile. Approximately 50–70 per cent of foetuses with a birth weight below tenth centile for gestational age are constitutionally small. If the baby is growing along its centile (its growth line on the ultrasound chart) and the fluid around the baby is normal then there is no need for worry. Otherwise you will be monitored more regularly and your care decided on the basis of scans and your and the baby's overall health.

If your baby is small at birth, he may be very hungry when he is born and he will soon make his weight up. A small baby is more at risk from low glucose and problems with temperature control and he will be watched carefully to see that he is putting on weight and thriving.

Excessive fluid – polyhydramnios

This is when there is an increased amount of amniotic fluid around your baby. Approximately half of such babies have no underlying cause and the pregnancy can carry on as normal as long as there is no effect on the baby's position.

The commonest other reason is diabetes in the mother. It can also occur with some anatomic defects (chest or gastrointestinal system), foetal anaemia and cardiac problems.

If your medical team sees increased fluid around the baby they will perform a glucose tolerance test and a detailed ultrasound will be done to exclude any anatomic problems. A test for viral infection and blood cell antibodies will be performed. The treatment depends on the underlying cause. Sometimes the excess fluid can be drained off by amniocentesis, and this may relieve some of the discomfort felt from the increase in size due to the extra fluid. You may also need to deliver early and if so you will be given steroid injections to help mature the baby's lungs.

Reduced fluid (oligohydramnios)

This can occur if your waters have broken. If this is the case you will be looked after according to how late you are in your pregnancy. If you are significantly under 24 weeks this is not good as reduced water around the baby affects how well the lungs develop. If you are at the end of your pregnancy then you may be able to have a normal labour, and if not you will be offered an induction. Sometimes you may have reduced fluid when the baby's growth has slowed, indicating that the placenta is not working as well as it should be. Very occasionally it can be due to a problem with the baby's gut or kidneys.

Breech presentation

The position of the baby is defined according to his lie in relation to the long axis of the uterus and his lowest (presenting) part.

Breech presentation is when his buttock is in the lower part of your uterus and his head is in the upper part of the uterus. One-quarter of babies are breech at 28 weeks, but as pregnancy progresses many of them turn, so really only between 3 and 4 per cent of pregnancies are breech by the end.

Risk factors include uterine malformations, small babies, excessive fluid around the baby, fibroids or placenta in the lower part of the uterus and multiple pregnancies. Rarely, a baby that has muscle weakness and is less active will be found in the breech position. Premature babies are much more likely to be breech.

If your baby is thought to be breech, then an ultrasound scan will be performed, which can confirm the position as well as the estimated foetal weight, the position of the placenta and the cord, if the baby's head is extended or flexed (drawn in) as well as any co-existent fibroids or pelvic masses that are obstructing the baby from being head down. This information can help plan how you deliver him.

There are three options for delivery:

- Caesarean section: Since 2000 it is generally recommended that women with breech babies have a Caesarean section at their due date. This is because the data from a large trial comparing vaginal delivery versus Caesarean section in breech babies noted that Caesarean section was safer.

- External cephalic version (ECV) is recommended to try to turn a baby from breech position to head down (cephalic) and this is done at between 37 and 38 weeks. The procedure can be done as long as there are no indications that vaginal delivery would be unsafe (for example, a low placenta). ECV is successful in between 50 and 60 per cent of cases, though there is a very small risk of foetal distress or the waters around the baby breaking and so bringing about a need for an emergency Caesarean section. If successful only about 5 per cent of babies revert to the breech position.

- Vaginal breech delivery: this should only be contemplated if you have been fully counselled and accept the additional risks to the baby of a breech delivery. This includes difficulty with delivery of the head once the bottom has delivered and the need to perform an emergency Caesarean section.

If your baby is lying sideways (transverse/oblique) and his head is not down towards the pelvis you will not be able to deliver vaginally. Risk factors are those of a breech baby.

Usually these babies turn or can be encouraged to turn using external cephalic version and then if they stay head down a vaginal delivery can take place.

If the waters break and if the baby is transverse, there is increased risk of the cord coming down before the baby (cord prolapse), and you will be warned about this (see also page 305). Some women are advised to stay in hospital if they are nearly at the end of their pregnancy and the baby is transverse. If the baby does not turn, then a Caesarean section is required.

Reduced foetal movements

You will usually feel the baby moving around 20 weeks into your pregnancy. To begin with the movements are just a flutter, but then they get more pronounced as the pregnancy progresses (see also page 153). Usually the baby will kick more than 10 times per day and so if you feel there are fewer than this or that there has been a decrease from what you normally feel, contact your GP the same day. If you feel no movements at all it is essential you go to the hospital that day. In the majority of cases there is absolutely nothing wrong with the baby and he will be monitored and you will be discharged. For some babies, the reduction in movements may indicate that the baby is getting stressed, which may necessitate an early delivery.

Rhesus disease

Rhesus is due to an incompatibility between the baby's and the mother's blood cells. At your booking visit blood will be taken to check what your blood group is, your rhesus status and red cell antibodies. On the surface of red blood cells there are a number of different proteins (antigens). If your baby has the rhesus antigen (rhesus positive) and you do not (rhesus negative) you may make antibodies to the baby's red cells. This does not usually affect your first pregnancy, but it can lead to the production of a powerful antibody response (sensitisation) in subsequent pregnancies if you have another rhesus-positive baby. You will produce more antibodies, and faster, and these will be able to cross the placenta to destroy the baby's blood cells, leading to severe anaemia in the baby.

To prevent development of antibodies in a first pregnancy an injection of Anti-D is given at 28 and 34 weeks, or one single dose at around 28 weeks. This will also be given if at any point there is bleeding, such as after the delivery or after operations such as for the termination of a pregnancy or a miscarriage, where a mother is rhesus negative and can still develop antibodies to a rhesus-positive baby. Anti-D destroys the foetal rhesus positive blood cells in the mother's circulation, so stopping antibodies being made by the mother.

Regular blood tests and scans will be done to check your antibody levels in any subsequent pregnancy. If the baby has severe anaemia he may be delivered early and sometimes a blood transfusion is given to him through the cord.

If you are rhesus negative your baby's father can be tested and if he is rhesus negative then your baby will be rhesus negative and there is no risk of the problem.

PART 3

Preparing for Life with Your Baby

11

Preparing Your Home

Getting your home ready to welcome your new baby is an enjoyable way of preparing for the birth, and it's good to think about this during your second trimester. You can start to imagine how life with your new baby is going to be while you are gathering together equipment and items for him. This process can be great fun, but it can also be a little bewildering since there is such a vast array of baby equipment available and you may not yet know quite what you really need. Added to this, friends and family may well offer you loads of advice about what they have found useful and advertising pressures may leave you feeling you need to spend out on expensive items that turn out to be not strictly necessary as time goes by.

It's a good idea to try to think beyond the baby stage and acquire furniture that you can adapt to be used later. For example you can buy chests of drawers that have removable changing-table tops. It's important to plan ahead for enough storage to adapt to your baby's rapidly changing needs. A few shelves stocked with basic storage boxes might do for the first tiny baby clothes and nappies, but in time you'll need to have hanging storage and cupboards for bigger clothes and shoes, plus plenty of toy storage.

If you can, try to do the following things before the baby is born – as this will free you up after the birth.

Things to do before the birth

- Get hold of as much nursery equipment in advance as you can. If you are buying new, items such as cots can sometimes take up to 12 weeks to be delivered. It's a good idea to install a big cot right from the time your baby is born so that he can get used to it gradually – and it means you only have to acquire one cot rather than several different versions (such as a Moses basket, crib and then the cot). You might find it a good idea to have a pram at the outset to use for daytime sleeps.

- Prepare the baby's bedclothes, muslins and towels by washing, ironing and airing them so that they are ready before the birth. You could make up the cot, Moses basket and pram (if you do decide to use these). Prepare as much as you can in the nursery so that it is ready beforehand. If your baby is sleeping in your own bedroom to begin with, get everything ready there.

- Stock up on supplies of the following baby essentials: cotton wool, baby oil, small-size nappies, muslin cloths, nappy and moisturising creams, baby wipes, soft sponges, a baby brush, bath oil and baby shampoo.

- Check that all the electrical equipment is working properly and that you have read the instructions. Learn how the steriliser works and how to assemble the feeding bottles, though you may not need these straight away.

- If you have the space, it might be a good idea to arrange a section of worktop in the kitchen where equipment can be sterilised and prepared and where the sterilising can be done. If possible, this should be directly below or above the cupboard where your baby's feeding equipment is kept.

- Buy in supplies of household essentials such as soap powder, cleaning materials and enough kitchen and toilet rolls to last at least six weeks – that way you won't have to go shopping for bulky household items in the early weeks. Alternatively, you can shop for these online and have them delivered.

- Cook and freeze batches of a large selection of healthy homemade meals. If you are breast-feeding, avoid buying ready-meals that may contain excessive amounts of additives and preservatives. However, it is a good idea to keep a few 'healthy' ready-meals in the freezer in case you run out of home-cooked food or don't feel like cooking – they are fine to have occasionally in the context of a well-balanced diet. Good-quality ready-meals, low in additives, are relatively easy to find.

- It is a good idea to buy in good supplies of dry goods such as tea, coffee and biscuits. You may find that you have extra visitors during the first month of your baby's life and you might want to offer them refreshments.

- If you are feeling really efficient and have the time, purchase gifts and cards for any important events that may be coming up. Though no one will be expecting you to send out birthday presents and cards while you are looking after a new baby, it might be a good idea to stock up on thank you cards for any baby gifts you may receive.

- Try to get any big household and garden jobs done in advance of your baby's birth.

● If you are breast-feeding and think you might find an electric milk-expressing machine useful, try to book one well in advance as they are much in demand. Ask your midwife for advice on how to do this.

Your baby's nursery

Most parents now have their babies sleeping in the same room as them during the night, at least for the first few weeks, and some adopt the co-sleeping method whereby baby and parents sleep in the same bed or the baby sleeps in a specially adjoining cot. The current advice from the Foundation for the Study of Infant Deaths (FSID) and the Department of Health is that your baby should sleep in the same room as you for all his sleeps until he is six months old. You should not share a bed with your baby if either you or your partner is a smoker of if you are under the influence of alcohol, illicit drugs or any medication that causes drowsiness.

It's a practical idea for the first few months, if your baby sleeps, is fed, changed and played with wherever you spend most of your time, but if it is feasible it is a good idea to have a separate room ready for your baby as soon as possible. Sometimes babies don't settle well when they are eventually transferred to an unfamiliar room, so it's a good strategy to use his own room as much as possible for nappy-changing, feeding and quiet play so that he gets used to being there. If you live in a flat, this routine is easier than if you have to go up and down stairs. But by getting your baby used to his own room from the outset, he will quickly enjoy being there and in a short time come to feel that it's his own peaceful space – invaluable in the months and years to come.

If your baby becomes upset, overtired or overstimulated, it is a real bonus to have a serene, cosy room where you can take him to calm down. Therefore using your baby's room in the early days will help him to make the transition from sleeping in your room to his own, once he reaches about six months of age.

Decorating your baby's room

If you have the time and resources it's nice to be able to redecorate your baby's room before he takes up residence – and you don't need to spend a fortune. If you keep things simple, you will not feel the need to keep changing the decor as your baby grows older and tires of nursery-style colours and decoration. For example, a room with walls, windows and bed linen covered in teddy bears and so on dates and starts to look babyish when your baby turns into a pre-school child, which happens all too rapidly. Therefore, it's probably best to opt for plain walls and the room can easily be brightened up with colourful accessories such as rugs, friezes and cushions; this makes it easy to adapt the room as your baby grows into a child and avoids the need to redecorate completely.

Your baby's cot

Many experts say that a 'proper' cot is not really necessary for newborns, as they seem more contented in a Moses basket or a small crib. These smaller pieces of equipment may make things easier for you if you are moving your baby from room to room with you during the day, but it is not clear whether babies really do sleep better in them. As your baby needs to get used to sleeping in the living area until he is six months old, it might be a better option to have an ordinary pram with a firm mattress for him to sleep in during the day. However, if you prefer to get your baby used to his big cot from day one, you could let him spend some time in his cot, having some quiet play and winding down after feeds. This means that you won't have a problem when he outgrows his Moses basket and starts to sleep the whole night in his big cot in his own room.

When you choose a cot, remember that it needs to serve as your baby's bed for at least two or three years, so it's important to get one that's solid enough to stand up to a toddler pulling himself up and perhaps bouncing up and down. And don't forget that even very young babies eventually start moving energetically around in their cot, putting its durability to the test. Perhaps the best plan is to choose a cot design that has flat bars rather than tubular ones – if your young baby presses his head against a tubular bar it could be quite painful.

Other things to consider when you are choosing a cot

● Look for a style that has two or three different base-height levels so that you can raise or lower the height according to the baby's age. Bending down to pick up a tiny baby can become very hard on your back.

● If they have drop sides they should be easy to pull up and down without making a noise that will disturb your sleeping baby. Some versions make it easy to do this one-handed. It's worth testing the model several times before you make a final purchasing decision.

● The cot should be large enough to accommodate a two-year-old child perfectly comfortably.

● All cots must comply with the recommendations set out by the British Standards Institute, Number BS1753. Bars must be no less than 2.5 cm (1 in) apart and no more than 6 cm (2½ in). When the mattress is in its lowest position, the maximum distance between that and the top of the cot should be 65 cm (26 in). There should be a gap of no more than 4 cm (1½ in) around the edge of the mattress.

● Buy the best possible quality of mattress that you can and never purchase a second-hand one. If you buy or are given a second-hand cot, it is vital to buy a new mattress to use with it. Foam mattresses tend to sink in the middle within a few months, so the type that gives the best support for growing babies is a 'natural cotton spring interior' type. All mattresses must comply with the British Safety Standards Numbers BS1877 and BS7177.

The bedding

It is important to make good choices when it comes to bedding. You may find yourself washing bedding on a daily basis and so it should all be made of 100 per cent white cotton, which can be boil-washed over and over again. You should avoid using baby duvets and cot quilts, pretty though they are, due to the risk of your young baby overheating or smothering. It's best to wait until he is at least one year old before you start to use one. If you want your baby's cot to have an attractive, colourful cover, make sure that it is made of 100 per cent cotton and that it does not contain a synthetic filling. If you like sewing, you can run up your own flat and draw sheets out of a large cotton double-bed sheet or lengths of purchased sheeting.

The changing station

Your life will be a lot simpler if you set up a proper nappy-changing station in your baby's room with everything you need stored in it, ready to hand. You might think of improvising with an ordinary table top, but be aware that your baby will soon be able to roll over – and even off – an ordinary table top, which will not have a fixed protective surround. Therefore it's worth investing in a proper changing station, which will comply with safety standards. When your baby has stopped using the changing station, you can transform it into useful bedroom storage. The best kind of changing station is a long unit containing drawers and a cupboard. The changing surface needs to be long enough to hold both the changing mat and the top-and-tail bowl. The drawers can hold all your baby's nightwear, vests and nappies, and muslins, and the cupboard can hold larger items, such as nappy packs and spare clothes.

Changing mats

You will need a changing mat or two to use on the changing station. Choose easy-clean plastic versions with well-padded sides. When your baby is very tiny it is best to place a hand towel on the mat or you can buy ready-made towelling changing-mat liners that are exactly the right size to fit it. Very young babies hate to be laid down on anything cold. It's well worth acquiring a travel changing mat to use when you are out and about – sometimes they are incorporated into changing bags, which hold everything you need when you go out.

The nursery chair

No matter how small your baby's room, it's a good idea to try to fit in a chair to make the room more relaxing. A sturdy, comfortable armchair is the best choice for feeding your baby in his own room and later perhaps for sitting in while you read him a story. A small sofa bed is a good idea to have, too. You can use it for feeding your baby in the early months and if you need to sleep in his room at any time, say, for example, if he is ill. If space in the room is limited, choose a chair with a straight back. It should be wide enough to allow space for you and your baby as he grows, and, ideally, the arms should be wide enough to support you while you are feeding him. Though pretty, rocking chairs, which are often sold as 'nursing chairs', are not necessarily a good idea. These can be dangerously unstable as your baby starts moving around and hauling himself up on things. It's also all too easy for your baby to get his fingers trapped under the rockers. When your baby is a newborn it can be tempting to rock him to sleep while holding him in a rocking chair, but this is not a good idea as it is one of the main reasons why babies develop poor sleeping habits – they learn to rely on the rocking motion to get themselves to sleep and can't then get to sleep on their own.

The nursery curtains

The curtains you choose for your baby's room should be full-length and fully lined with blackout lining so that you can get the room really dark – this will help to get him into a good sleep routine. Research has shown that chemicals in the brain alter in the dark, conditioning the body for sleep, so it makes good sense to make the room as dark as possible. Fix the curtains to a track that fits flush along the top of the window. It's a good idea if curtains have a deep, matching pelmet that is also lined with blackout lining, so that all light can be excluded from the room. There should be no gaps between the sides of the curtains and the window frame; even the smallest chink of light can be enough to wake a baby too early in the morning. For the same reason, avoid installing curtain poles – the light will stream through the gap at the top. As time goes by and your baby gets older, he may not be able to go back to sleep if he is woken by bright early-morning sun in summer, or by bright street lights in winter.

Is the room dark enough?

A good test to see whether the room is dark enough is to turn all lights off, close the curtains and see whether you can see another person standing on the other side of the room.

Carpets and floor coverings

It's a good idea to put a fully fitted carpet into your baby's room and this is a better choice than a rug, which you might accidentally trip over in dim light. Choose one that is treated with a stain-guard so that you don't have to worry about the odd spill, and avoid having one that is either very dark or bright in colour – these may show the dirt more easily.

Lighting in your baby's room

Rather than having a constantly bright central light in your baby's room, you can quickly calm the lighting by installing a dimmer switch. When your baby is still little, lowering the lights when settling him is a very good way of signalling to him that it's time for sleep. He will soon get the message, so it's worth starting the habit early. If you don't want to install a permanent fitting you can buy a small plug-in nightlight that fits any normal 13-amp electrical socket – this will create a soothing low light in the room while you are putting him to bed. However, remember to turn it off when it's time for your baby to go to sleep.

Baby equipment you will need

If this is your first pregnancy, it may be tempting to go for the most up-to-date equipment you can afford. However, it's important to look ahead and avoid spending out on gimmicky things that you may not really need. You can make some really significant savings at a very costly time by buying second-hand rather than new and there are bargains to be found at car boot sales, charity shops and online auction sites; some items are brand new or hardly used. However, it is important that second-hand items comply with the latest safety standards. You might think that you're somehow letting your baby down by buying second-hand, but as long as he is warm, safe and comfortable, he will be perfectly happy.

Moses basket or small crib

A Moses basket is not really an essential piece of equipment, though it can be convenient for carrying around your home in the very early days of your baby's life. Even the cheapest kind, with its own stand, can be pricey and, pretty though cribs are, bear in mind that your baby will outgrow it within six weeks and need to move into the big cot. If your budget is limited, perhaps you could borrow one from a friend, though you will still need to buy a new mattress for it. The Foundation for the Study of Infant Deaths (FSID) strongly recommends that you do so. All new mattresses should carry the BSI number BS1877 and BS7177.

A crib is really a small version of a big cot. Some styles come on rockers or on wheels, which can be convenient. Cribs are longer than a Moses basket, but they are not really any more practical. You can also buy 'bassinettes', which come without bars, but with a storage tray below and wheels for easy movement. Because babies are now put down to sleep on their backs to reduce the risk of sudden infant death syndrome (SIDS), narrow cribs may not be a good idea. This is because babies sleeping on their backs can wake themselves up several times a night if the crib is not wide enough for them to sleep with their arms stretched out fully, and they may get their hands caught between the bars.

Pram or buggy

The old-style traditional pram tends to be quite pricey and is perhaps not entirely suitable for modern life, where you may need to use a car a lot. However, these prams are perfect if you want to put your newborn baby to sleep in it during the day indoors. For going out, most parents find it more practical to choose one of the other, more compact, types of baby transport. When you choose a pram, carry-cot or buggy, it is important to plan for, according to FSID guidelines, your baby sleeping in it during the day until he is six months old.

The buggy

Think hard about choosing a buggy. Many parents end up buying different buggies for their baby's various stages – or even one for the car and one for the house – because the first buggy they bought turns out to be too big to go in the car boot. You can save a lot of trouble and expense by buying one that is suitable for all your needs from birth to about age three. The buggy needs to be the right height for you to push (so if you are tall, check that you don't have to bend down to manipulate the buggy), and is easily manoeuvrable. You also need to think about your environment and lifestyle. If you do a lot of driving, for example, it is important to choose a buggy that you can fold up easily and which is not too heavy to lift in and out of the boot. There are now very good lightweight buggies available that can recline flat and are suitable for a newborn baby. They come with a hood and apron to give the baby good protection in bad weather. Beware of 'colour-coding' (blue for boys and pink for girls), but rather buy one in a colour that is gender-neutral. You can then perhaps use it for another baby, who may be of the other sex. There are plenty of colours to choose from that suit both sexes.

Travel system

A good and popular option is a 'three-in-one' travel system, which is a transporter that can be used with a carry-cot when your baby is newborn and with a buggy-type seat when he is a little older. This may be a very good choice if you intend to walk directly from home without using a car or public transport. The third choice is a heavier-weight version of the light buggy, which reclines flat for a newborn and usually comes with a mattress.

Swivel wheels

If you live in a town or need to wheel your baby in confined spaces such as supermarket aisles, swivel wheels are a big plus. They make turning the buggy or pram around tight corners so much easier compared to those with set wheels.

Try the buggy out first

Whichever type of buggy you choose, practise putting it up and down a few times, and try lifting it on to a surface in the shop to get an idea of how easy it is going to be to put it into the car. Try pushing it around the shop to check whether the handle height is comfortable – some buggies come with adjustable-height handles.

Car seat

You will need to have a car seat ready-installed to bring your baby home from hospital and it is now the law that all babies must travel in them, whatever their age. It is now normal practice for a midwife to accompany you to your car when you are discharged from hospital to check that you have a baby seat installed properly.

You must always put your baby into his car seat, no matter how short your journey. Never be tempted to travel holding your baby in your arms as, in the event of a collision or emergency stop, it would be impossible to keep hold of him. If your car is fitted with emergency air bags, unless these have been adequately disabled, you should not fit the baby seat into the front seat. Last, but not least, choose the best-quality baby seat you can afford.

Baby bath

A small baby bath is an item that is not absolutely essential to have. Like the Moses basket, babies outgrow the small bath very quickly. If you want to experiment with not having one first, try bathing your newborn in an ordinary hand basin or even try him out in the big bath using a special baby bath seat. Your baby lies supported on a slight slope, leaving you with both hands free to wash him and you may find this more practical in the early days and weeks.

If you want to use a special baby bath, try a version that fits across or inside the big bath. This makes filling and emptying easy. Another design to investigate is a bath that is incorporated in a changing station. However, research the design thoroughly before you buy as some are more difficult to use and empty than others.

Baby monitor

Baby monitors can be extremely useful and save a lot of parental anxiety. There is a wide range to choose from: some just monitor sounds, while others can sense movement too. A mobile version may suit you better than a plug-in type as it allows you to move freely around your home, including areas such as the bathroom. There is a growing body of scientific evidence to suggest that digital (or DECT) monitors expose babies to more pulsing microwave radiation than mobile phone base station masts. For this reason, it is better to choose an analogue baby monitor.

Baby sling

Some parents swear by slings as they allow them to move around while carrying their baby and they can have their hands free at the same time. This is ideal, for example, if you are on public transport and need to hold on to other children or shopping. However, if you are following a specific sleep routine with your baby, you may find that your baby falls asleep the moment he is put into a sling, which may then disrupt his sleep pattern, causing him to wake more than usual at night. But as your baby gets bigger, you may find that a sling is a very useful way to carry him around, especially when he is old enough to face forwards and see the world go by.

Baby chair

You may find that you can use your baby's car seat in the house for your baby to sit in during the day. But having a second seat for him can be a bonus as it saves having to move seats from car to home and back every time.

Baby seats come in many different styles. Some are rigid, though you can adjust the seat positions, and they have a base that can either remain stable or be set to rocking mode. Another type is known as a 'bouncy chair', which is made of a lightweight fabric-covered frame designed to bounce slightly as the baby moves. Babies aged over two months seem to enjoy them, but they are not really suitable for newborns as they can make them feel insecure. Always make sure that your baby is securely strapped into his chair and never leave him unattended in it. Choose the position of the chair carefully. You should always place it on the floor – well away from draughts – and never put him on a table or worktop. The movement of the baby in the chair can easily shift the chair to the edge of the surface and he could fall off.

Playpen

Playpens are sometimes frowned upon, but they can be very useful at times. Some parents feel that they stop a mobile baby freely exploring his environment and while it's true that you should not leave your baby in a playpen for long spells, they can enable your baby to be safe when you have to do something else such as go to the loo or answer the door. If you do decide to use a playpen, it's a good idea to get your baby used to it as young as possible. You can use a travel cot as a small playpen, but if you have the space, the square, wooden type, which is larger and would enable your baby to pull himself up and move around when he reaches the right age, is perhaps the better option. Whichever you choose, place the playpen out of reach of hazards such as radiators, curtains and trailing electrical flexes. Don't be tempted to hang toys on pieces of string or cord in the playpen, as these could be hazardous if your baby got tangled in them.

Breast-feeding accessories

Nursing bra

These are special bras with cups that you can either unhook or unzip to make breast-feeding more convenient. You don't have to remove it to feed your baby. It is important that whatever style of bra you choose fits well, so it's a good idea to be professionally measured before you buy. Bear in mind, also, that your breasts may change in size over the months, so you may need to be measured several times. A good nursing bra should preferably be made of cotton for comfort, have wide, adjustable shoulder straps to provide maximum support and should not press tightly against your nipples, as this can cause your milk ducts to become blocked. You could just buy two before your baby is born and if they are still comfortable after your milk has come in, you could perhaps buy two more.

Breast pads

These pads absorb any leaks in between feeds. When you first start breast-feeding you will probably use a lot of breast pads, as they need to be changed every time you breast-feed. Many women prefer the circular style, contoured to fit the breasts, but you can experiment with different types until you find the best ones for you. Sometimes the more expensive ones offer better absorbency, so these may work out better value in the long run.

Nursing pillow

These special pillows are a real asset when you are breast-feeding as they help support your back, which is vital if you are to feed your baby comfortably and successfully. Nursing pillows are shaped to fit around your waist, so that your baby can be raised to the correct height for feeding. At other times these cushions are useful for propping your baby up and they make an excellent back support when he is learning to sit up. If you decide to buy one, make sure it has a removable, machine-washable cover.

Nipple creams and sprays

These creams and sprays are used to care for the breasts and help to relieve any pain you may experience when you breast-feed. However, the main cause of any pain is usually as a result of your baby not being latched on properly. If you experience pain either during or after feeding, consult your health visitor or breast-feeding counsellor for advice before purchasing a cream or spray as there may be another reason for the pain or other ways to solve the problem. To care for your breasts normally, simply rub your nipples with a little breast milk after each feed and, if possible, allow them to air-dry.

Electric breast milk expressing machine

There are many reasons why you might want to use an electric breast pump: you may be returning to work or just going out for the evening and want your baby to have your breast milk in your absence. Or your partner may want to be involved in feeding his baby. Whatever your reasons, a breast pump expresses the milk fast and encourages it to keep flowing. This may help breast-feeding to be more successful for you and your baby.

In the early days of your baby's life, when you are producing more milk than your baby may need (especially first thing in the morning), it can be expressed quickly and stored in the fridge or freezer to be used as a top-up later in the day when you may be tired and your milk supply is low. Low milk supply may be one of the main reasons why many babies are restless and find it hard to settle after their evening bath.

So if you want to breast-feed and get your baby into a routine, an electric pump will be a great asset. Do not be tempted by one of the smaller hand versions, which can be so inefficient as to put many women off expressing at all.

You can store expressed milk in the fridge for up to 24 hours or in the freezer for one month. Specially designed, pre-sterilised bags are an ideal way to store the milk and are available from chemists or baby departments in larger stores.

Bottle-feeding accessories

Feeding bottles

If you are breast-feeding your baby successfully, you may assume that you won't need bottles now or ever. Many breast-feeding counsellors advise against newborns being given any bottle, even of expressed milk, claiming that it creates 'nipple confusion' in the baby and reduces his desire to suck at the breast, leading to a weaker milk supply and the mother even eventually having to give up breast-feeding. It's certainly true that many women do give up breast-feeding because they are exhausted by 'demand feeding', which could happen several times a night in the early days.

Introducing just one bottle

One possible solution is to give your baby a bottle of either expressed milk or formula milk from the first week, introducing it by the fourth week at the latest. Your baby can be given this one bottle either last thing at night or during the night by your partner, so that you can sleep for several hours undisturbed. This, in turn, is likely to make you more able to cope with breast-feeding and it is unlikely that your baby will reject the breast or become confused between your nipple and the bottle teat (though this could happen if, early on, your baby is offered more than one bottle a day).

Other good reasons for getting your baby used to a single bottle are: firstly, it gives you a little flexibility and freedom – you don't have to be with him every hour of the day; secondly, the problem of introducing bottles later to an exclusively breast-fed baby doesn't crop up; and thirdly, it gives your baby's father a great chance to get involved in feeding his baby and bond with him more fully.

Styles of bottle

Bottles come in all shapes and sizes, but the wide-necked variety is highly recommended because cleaning and filling is easier. Look for bottles that are free of Bisphenol A (BPA) as some scientists believe that this chemical, which is commonly found in clear plastic feeding bottles, can actually leach out into the milk.

Start off by using a newborn teat, which will have a slow flow, encouraging your baby to work as hard during feeding from the bottle as when he is breast-feeding. However, using a teat that is too slow can lead to problems such as wind, so see what your baby prefers and switch over to a faster-flowing teat if he seems to be finding it tricky. This may happen as early as three weeks, but usually takes place when he is around eight weeks old.

Exclusive bottle-feeding

If your baby is likely to take all his milk from a bottle, it is important that the risk of developing colic or wind is kept to a minimum and this can be done by using a wide-necked bottle. The teat is designed to be flexible, allowing the baby to suckle as he would at the breast. Later on, you can adapt the wide-necked bottles to become feeding beakers by adding soft spouts and handles. If your baby is being exclusively bottle-fed, start off with five 240 ml (8 oz) bottles and three 120 ml (4 oz) bottles.

Teats and brushes

To begin with, use a slow-flow teat designed for newborns – these are usually sold with most feeding bottles. By eight weeks most babies feed better from a medium-flow teat, so it's a good idea to stock up on these at the outset so that you have them to hand when you need them.

It's extremely important to clean baby bottles thoroughly, so choose a brush with an extra-long handle so that you can use more force when cleaning. The easiest way to clean a teat is by using your forefinger. However, if you have extra-long nails, it may be worthwhile investing in a special teat brush, although you have to be careful as they can damage the teat hole, and you'll have to replace teats more frequently.

The sterilising process

You might find it easier to keep track of what is sterilised and what is not if you wash and sterilise all the used bottles at once. Find a suitable place to keep the rinsed-out bottles and teats until you are ready to sterilise them. A large bowl, either stainless steel or plastic, is ideal. If it has a lid, this is even better.

The steriliser

Whether you are breast- or bottle-feeding, or both, it is vital that all bottles and expressing equipment are sterilised thoroughly. You can choose from three main methods: boiling items for 10 minutes in a large pan; soaking items in a sterilising solution (available from chemists) for two hours and rinsing with boiling water; or using an electric steam steriliser. The easiest, most efficient and most effective method is the steam steriliser, and it is well worth purchasing one (you will need to sterilise all your baby's feeding equipment and other items that go into his mouth, such as teething rings and rattles, until he is one year old). Don't be tempted to purchase a microwave version, since these units hold fewer bottles and could be very inconvenient when you need to use the microwave for other things.

Kettle

This ordinary item of kitchen equipment is essential for making up feeds, so your kettle should be efficient and large enough to boil up a decent amount of water in one go. If you bottle-feed your baby formula right from the beginning you will quickly become an expert in making up feeds. Therefore you might want to buy a second kettle. The water for making up the formula must be fresh, boiled only once and cooled before you add the powder. Therefore, it's inconvenient if someone boils the kettle again while you are waiting for your water to cool – though, of course, you could decant the cooling water.

Bottle insulator

If you do a lot of travelling or want to make up night feeds quickly, a bottle insulator could prove very helpful. This is a special type of

Thermos designed to keep bottles of boiled water warm. When you buy a bottle insulator, choose a small, plastic, three-sectioned container. You can then put the required amount of formula for three different feeds into each section, which means that you don't have to carry a tin of formula around.

Newborn clothes

The dazzling array of baby clothes on display in the shops is both tempting and overwhelming. It can be fun choosing sweet little things for your baby, but it pays to be cautious as you can end up spending unnecessarily. Newborn babies grow very fast and outgrow most first-size clothes after just a month, unless they were small at birth. However, you will need to have plenty of clothes in order to change your baby fairly frequently – sometimes several times a day – but if you have too many clothes, you may find that you hardly get any wear out of them and some will be barely used. You'll probably need to acquire a new set of clothes at least three times in the first year, and this could prove expensive. Therefore it's best to buy only the basics before your baby's birth and you may be lucky enough to be given baby clothes by friends and relatives when your baby arrives.

When it comes to choosing baby clothes for the first month of your baby's life, it's best to avoid buying anything that's too brightly coloured, for example, vests or sleepwear. It can be very difficult to get rid of stubborn stains by washing at any temperature less than 60°C and some items might be damaged by a hot wash. Brightly coloured garments will soon fade if you wash them frequently at this temperature, so it's probably best to stick to whites and pastels and just reserve brighter shades for the outer garments, which don't need to be washed so often.

As a first principle, you are better off keeping your baby's clothing as simple as possible for the first month and it makes good sense to dress your baby in little white vests and white baby-grows in the early days – laundry is far more straightforward when you can put everything in to be washed at the same time, without worrying about different colours and fabrics. It's worth investing in a tumble-dryer so that you do not have to iron.

Here is a basic list of the items you require for the first two months of your baby's life. However, it's probably best not to remove packaging or tags before you try them on, in case you have to take any items back to the shop – your baby may be larger or smaller than the typical birth size.

Essential baby clothing basics

- 6–8 vests

- 2–3 pairs of socks

- 4–6 nightdresses or sleep suits

- 2 hats

- 4–6 daytime outfits

- 2 pairs of mittens

- 2–3 cardigans

- 3 shawls

- 1 snowsuit (for a winter baby)

- 1 jacket

Vests

Except in extremely hot weather, you need to put your newborn baby into a vest, both winter and summer. Choose 100 per cent cotton – it's best next to your baby's delicate skin and it retains its snowy appearance even after numerous washes. Choose plain white or white with a pale-coloured pattern. A good style of vest to buy is a 'body suit', which poppers under your baby's crotch, with short sleeves and an envelope-style neckline so that you can ease it over his head without it getting caught.

Nightwear

A good choice for your new baby's sleepwear are the all-in-one sleep suits, or 'baby-grows', which are warm and snug. You may already be dressing him in these during the day. Because they are all-in-one they save time on laundry – you only have to wash one item. The only downside is that they can be awkward if you have to manipulate your sleepy baby out of one to change his nappy at night. So some parents opt for nightdresses or 'bundlers', which have no fastenings, at least for the early weeks. Choose 100 per cent cotton and a simple design that doesn't have ties anywhere – your baby could get caught up in them and they could be a choking hazard. You can buy baby 'grobags', which are suitable when your baby is a few weeks old. These are essentially padded sleeping bags, which prevent the risk of overheating from using too much bedding. In addition, the bedding cannot accidentally slip over the baby's head. And because the baby's feet and legs are inside the bag, they cannot get stuck between cot bars.

Daytime outfits

For the first two months or so after the birth, you will probably find that the easiest items for your baby to wear are baby-grows.

Try to select pure cotton and choose a style that opens up either across the back or up the legs and under the crotch. This will mean that you don't need to undress your baby completely when it comes to changing his nappy. Dungaree-style garments in soft, stretchy fabrics, without feet and with matching T-shirts, are also useful. They will last a bit longer as your baby grows, and it's easy enough to change the tops if necessary. Velour is an ideal fabric for very young babies – avoid choosing stiff cottons or denim, which can restrict the baby's movements.

Cardigans

If yours is a summer baby, you probably only need two cardigans, ideally made from cotton, but winter babies need at least three, preferably made from real wool. If you dress your baby with cotton next to his skin, the wool will not irritate it. Choose as simple a design as possible.

Socks

Choose simple socks in cotton or wool. Don't be tempted by complicated styles with ribbons, or any kind of 'shoe' style, however sweet and appealing, as they could harm your baby's delicate bones, which are still soft. Socks and bootees should fit snugly, but not be too tight. The 'roll top' style of sock is good, as it is less likely to fall off.

Hats

Babies' heads are very vulnerable and you should put a hat on your baby whenever you take him outside – whatever the season or the weather. Some tiny newborns need a hat indoors as some homes are draughty. For summer, he should wear a cotton hat with a wide brim to protect his head and face from the sun. If possible, the brim should go all the way around, shading the back of his neck. In spring and autumn, knitted cotton hats are fine for cooler days. Don't be tempted to dress him in a peaked cap, which has no protection for the neck. During the winter, or on very cold days, opt for a warm wool or fleece hat lined with cotton. If it is not cotton-lined, you can put a thin cotton hat underneath to protect his sensitive skin.

Mittens

Small babies hate having their hands covered, as they use them extensively to touch, feel and explore, but sometimes it is essential if your baby tends to scratch himself with his sharp nails. You could try fine cotton 'scratch mitts', which are made for this purpose. In very cold weather dress your baby in woollen or fleece mitts, but put cotton ones underneath if he has sensitive skin.

Swaddling using a shawl or blanket

During the early weeks babies tend to sleep better when they are swaddled snugly. You can use a blanket or a shawl for this, though it should be made of lightweight, pure cotton that is slightly stretchy. Swaddle your baby in just one layer, otherwise he might get overheated, and when he is sleeping while swaddled, reduce the number of blankets you put on him in the cot. By the time he is six weeks old you can start getting your baby used to being half-swaddled, just under the arms, so that his hands are free. Overheating is thought to be a major factor in cot death and it's all too easy to wrap your baby up too warmly – cot death rates peak between two and four months of age. Check that you are not putting too many layers on your baby and that the room temperature is always between 16–20°C (60–68°F), as recommended by the Foundation for the Study of Infant Deaths.

Snowsuits and jackets

It's a good idea to always buy outer garments at least two sizes too big for your baby, as this allows plenty of room for growth (snowsuits are not always cheap). Avoid choosing complicated designs with fur around the hood or toggles, which could pose a choking hazard – instead go for an easy-care washable fabric and a plain style. For tiny babies, poppers may be a better choice of fastening than a zip, which can easily dig into your baby's chin. However, whichever style of fastening you choose, ensure that it undoes all the way down, so that you can change your baby's nappy easily.

You will find that having a lightweight jacket will be useful at any time of the year – great for both chilly summer and spring days and milder winter days.

Moving house

When you know you are expecting a new baby and your family is about to increase in size, your home might suddenly seem a little too cramped. Moving house can be stressful, so now is not an ideal time to move, but it's not impossible and it may be something you have little choice about. Think carefully about what sort of home you want – it might help to make a checklist of the issues that might be important at this stage.

What sort of new home?

Perhaps you're moving from a small flat to a larger one or into a house. Consider the following:

- Two or more bedrooms?

- A garden or patio?

- Plenty of storage space, such as an attic or cellar, wardrobes and fitted cupboards?

- No steps or minimum number of steps or a lift to your front door? This will make manipulating a buggy far easier.

- A wide hallway? You won't have to fold up the buggy all the time – and there'll be more space for changing bags, shopping, shoes and coats.

- A spacious kitchen that includes a dining area?

- Door into the garden? Think ahead. If you can keep an eye on small children playing in the garden while you're in the kitchen, this will make life easier and more enjoyable.

Also think carefully about:

- How near are your extended family and friends?

- Are there toddler groups, playgroups and nurseries nearby?

- Is there a good choice of local schools?

- Is there public transport nearby?

- Are there parks, green spaces and leisure centres?

- Are there local doctors' surgeries, dentists and clinics?

- Where is the nearest accident and emergency department?

- Are there shops nearby?

Your family

If you have any choice about where you live, having parents or other relatives who can babysit is a real plus. This will give you a little freedom to have an affordable social life in the early years and it's also reassuring to be reasonably close to your parents for when they need you to help them. Also, your kids will be able to bond with their relatives, which is much harder if there is distance between you.

Schools

If this is your first baby, choosing a school may seem to be a long way off. However, schools are often at the top of people's lists when they move house and the time soon flies by. If your family is very young, you might only be thinking about local nurseries and primaries at this point, but it may be worth thinking about secondary schools at this stage too. That way you can avoid moving again in a few years' time and you can maintain the friendships and bonds forged in the early stages of your child's life.

Public transport

Are you considering moving from an urban to a rural setting? This can be great for young children, but think hard about whether this is what you really want to do yourself. If you're not within walking distance of reliable public transport, you can end up spending a lot of time driving – to schools, childcare, after-school activities, play dates, surgeries, to the shops and, of course, to work.

Parks and leisure centres

Safe green spaces with good play areas, and a leisure centre with a pool and other child-friendly facilities are well worth considering. Thinking of things to do with small children on long winter weekends is a recurrent challenge, and centres with ball-pits and soft-play areas can be a real plus.

Medical services

How close will you be to a maternity unit, an accident and emergency unit, a hospital with a special care baby unit? The NHS website (see Resources, page 328) has a facility (in the NHS Choices section) that allows you to see which services individual hospitals offer and how other patients have rated them. When you have young children, the GP, practice nurse and your local A&E or minor injuries unit may become very familiar, so being relatively close is important. Even if you guard against all the commonest accidents, they do happen and if your child eventually plays sports, sports injuries are a fact of life.

Renovation

If you are already happy with your good-sized home, but it needs to stretch to accommodate your expanding family, you could think about having a loft conversion done or a kitchen extension added. However, remember that major renovation projects and small children or babies are not a good combination, so you might need to move out temporarily.

If there is space and the opportunity, add more storage than you think you will need, and put in an extra bathroom or shower room if you have the space. A family bathroom is great while kids are little, but later on you'll need more bathroom facilities such as an extra shower.

12

Your Changing Relationships

Pregnancy can be a fantastic experience, bringing you closer to your partner and helping you both to discover new things to love about each other that perhaps you never noticed before. However, it would be unhelpful to think that such a seismic change to your lives together will not also come with new challenges and tensions.

Of course, it's not just your relationship with your partner that will change. Your new pregnancy is bound to affect the relationships you have with your friends, parents, siblings and in-laws.

With a little advice, guidance and understanding you can easily overcome any difficulties, ensuring that the impact your pregnancy has on your relationships is a positive one and that this is the wonderfully bonding time it should be for you all.

Tending your relationship with your partner

If you have both been wanting a baby for some time, the moment you tell your partner that you are expecting his child is an amazing one that you'll remember forever. However, the first few weeks after you discover you're pregnant can also be some of the most challenging. You'll feel elation, particularly if this is a long-sought-after pregnancy, and you and your partner will enjoy sharing this wonderful secret. However, it is also only natural that you will be feeling fears and doubts and these might be exacerbated by the hormonal changes you will be experiencing and the nausea and exhaustion you might suddenly be feeling. If your pregnancy is not common knowledge yet, there will be few people other than your partner with whom you can share your feelings.

Good communication

This time is an excellent opportunity to set up good communication habits with your partner that will strengthen your relationship throughout pregnancy and into parenthood. Keep in mind that you are going through this pregnancy together as a couple, rather than as individuals. With such huge changes taking place in your lives it's vital that you both get on board and make the transition together. Otherwise there's a risk that one of you will feel very enthusiastic about the pregnancy and the prospect of being a parent, while the other feels as if they are being left behind, perhaps yearning for your old child-free life and the way your relationship used to be. If you can approach pregnancy and parenthood as a team it will be one of the most rewarding and bonding times in your relationship.

The first opportunity to start the bonding process is immediately after you discover you're pregnant. You will both be experiencing a wide range of emotions, positive and negative, so be open with each other and discuss them. This will help reassure you both that you are not alone in your feelings and it will help you to bond.

Your partner's feelings

If you find at times that your partner seems to have more worries about impending parenthood than you do, don't interpret this negatively. It simply means that's he is taking the very real responsibilities of becoming a father seriously and it will probably only be a matter of weeks before you swap positions and he will be the one who is comforting you through your anxieties.

If your partner does not seem to want to discuss his feelings, ask him if he can identify with any of the issues on pages 30–1 and let him know if any of them are worrying you. You might also think about using a counselling service like Relate (see Resources, page 331). Sometimes an objective person can help you see things more clearly.

Once you've discussed your feelings and concerns about your pregnancy with your partner, the next step is to help him feel as involved in the pregnancy as possible. At this stage you might well be resenting the fact that all the physical changes of pregnancy are happening to you while he seems unaffected and carries on his life as normal. But this does also mean that he might feel left out of the process.

Getting your partner to feel that he is involved in the pregnancy is another great opportunity to help you both feel you can go through this change together.

How your partner can become involved

- Read up on pregnancy together. Perhaps suggest that he reads the same books that you're reading or perhaps others, too, and that he fills you in on what they say. Understanding the science behind what is going on in your body will help him feel more informed and less alienated by what's happening. He may well enjoy becoming an 'expert' on the subject. Although it may be tempting, resist the urge to put him down for not knowing enough and don't act as though you have superior knowledge – a free exchange of information will benefit both of you.

- Plan to attend antenatal classes together. This will make him feel well informed. He'll be able to ask questions and have a chance to meet other dads-to-be.

- Help him have as much contact with his unborn baby as possible. The moment you first feel your child moving inside you is a truly bonding experience, but remember that fathers don't get to experience this directly. So encourage your partner to feel the baby's movements with his hand, and ask him to come to ultrasound scans with you so that he can see his child on screen. Get him to listen to the baby's heartbeat (he can do this by placing his ear on your bump from 30 weeks onwards). You could even encourage him to read or sing to the baby if he's keen. Babies can often recognise their father's lower-pitched voice more easily than their mother's and, if nothing else, it will be an entertaining and bonding experience for both of you.

- Get him to massage your back, feet and legs. It will provide you with a very relaxing experience, he'll enjoy being able help you and it will be a bonding experience for you both.

- When it's time, put him in charge of getting the baby's room ready. It will be a helpful thing to do anyway, especially in the later stages of pregnancy, when you are feeling tired. It will help him feel truly valued.

- Ask him to shop/cook/help around the house more than usual. Explain how helpful it will be to you if he takes more of these tasks on and tell him exactly what he could do that would be most useful.

- Exercise together. Go for a walk or a swim together. You'll both feel better for it and it will give you a chance to spend quality time together.

- When the time comes, write your birth plan (see page 128) together. It's hard to feel sympathetic about any fears your partner might be feeling about your baby's birth, given that you are the one who is having to go through it, but bear in mind that he probably is feeling at least some anxiety. He may be afraid of seeing you in pain and not rising to the occasion and supporting you in the best way possible. Knowing exactly how you'd like the birth to go will help you both overcome your worries – and if he is going to be your birth partner he will need to be well acquainted with what you'd like to happen.

Advice for dads-to-be

Although becoming a father for the first time may be one of the most wonderful experiences of your life, it is only natural to have a few anxieties and doubts. However, such feelings simply show that you are taking your new role and the responsibilities that come with it seriously and this bodes well for you in becoming a wonderful father.

The moment you first discover that your partner is expecting, when you first announce the news to family and friends and when you start to see your partner's emerging bump – these are all times when it is only normal to feel a fresh flush of concerns creeping into your mind. Most of the time, this is simply because impending fatherhood suddenly feels more 'real'.

Discussing feelings

It is vital that you discuss your feelings, both positive and negative, with your partner. Even if she seems thrilled to be pregnant you'll be amazed at how many anxieties are shared by both of you. Use the list on pages 30–1, which details the most common worries experienced by parents-to-be, to reassure yourself that your fears really are normal. You can instigate a discussion with your partner about what is on your mind. Tell her which of the thoughts on the list apply to you and ask her which have been worrying her.

Feeling left out

As your baby begins to grow, your partner will start to feel changes in her body and it's all too easy for you to feel a little left out. She is getting direct experience of her approaching parenthood and her life is already changing, while your life remains very much the same. You may also feel pushed out by female family members, who may seem to have a better understanding of what's happening than you do and may even want to keep the conversation women-only. There are also doctors who might choose to direct questions to just your partner rather than to both of you.

It is very important at this point that you don't simply take a back seat during the pregnancy. This is your child and you have more right than most to be involved in the pregnancy. Taking a back seat risks allowing a gulf to build between you and your partner. She may embrace the pregnancy and subsequent parenthood, leaving you feeling abandoned and detached from your new way of life, mourning the way things used to be.

Getting involved

Becoming involved in the pregnancy is very easy and can be hugely rewarding. There are few things more amazing than feeling your child kick under your hand for the first time. And there are few things more bonding than the gratitude your partner will express when you offer her a foot massage at the end of a long day. See below for a list of the ways you, as a potential father, can become more involved with your partner's pregnancy. You might find some of the ideas more satisfying and enjoyable than others, but it is well worth giving them a try.

Your role of a father-to-be during your partner's pregnancy is not to be underestimated. You will usually be her primary support, particularly if your extended family does not live nearby. This kind of support is key to her well-being and makes you invaluable to her.

Pregnancy can be a wonderfully bonding time for a couple. However, your partner's exhaustion, possible morning sickness and her fluctuating hormones may mean that this time will present its challenges. The list below includes tips and suggestions, which should help you to overcome them.

Tips for prospective fathers

- Keep communication between you open. It may be that your partner is acting in a certain way because she has something on her mind, or if something is worrying you, then this may be affecting your behaviour more than you realise. If you discuss how you feel it will benefit you both.

- Remember that pregnancy hormones don't remain there forever. Even if your partner is usually an even-tempered person, it's likely that during pregnancy her emotions will be up and down, causing her to veer between tears, anger and elation all in a short time. Remember that she can't always help this, and that it can be just as bewildering for her as it is for you. She's enduring this to bring your child into the world and once the nine months are up she will return to being the balanced person you first fell in love with.

- Be prepared for your sex life to become erratic. During the first few months of pregnancy, when she's possibly suffering with morning sickness, she may go off the idea of sex altogether, but then in the second trimester she might not be able to keep her hands off you! When a woman is pregnant, her sexual urges are likely to become as unpredictable as her emotions. Remember that this is simply a hormonal reaction to pregnancy. Reassure her that even though her body is changing you still find her attractive, enjoy the times she does want to have sex, and when she doesn't remember that you can always show affection by cuddling, kissing or caressing each other.

- Remind her that you still find her attractive. This is so important. On top of being on a hormonal roller coaster, your partner is also dealing with her body changing in ways she may not have anticipated. Reassuring her that you still find her beautiful will make her feel happier and strengthen your relationship.

- Expect her to want to spend more time with her mother. Mothers and daughters often find pregnancy a very bonding time. Encourage this and don't feel threatened if they want to spend time together without you.

- If you don't know what to do to help, ask. If your partner is suffering from a bad bout of morning sickness or is feeling melancholy for no apparent reason you may feel that there's nothing you can do. At these times there's no harm in asking. There might be something she'd like you to do and, if not, she'll feel better because you have shown that you care.

- Help around the house a bit more than you usually do. Men often don't realise quite how much partners appreciate this. If she's feeling overwhelmed and exhausted, discovering that you've brought home a take-away or unloaded the dishwasher can be a real boost. Try to anticipate what needs doing, but if you're not sure just ask.

- Find a 'pub buddy'. Having a friend, particularly if he is a father himself, who you can talk to when things are becoming a bit too much can be very helpful. Simply getting out of the house (not necessarily to the pub) and offloading to a friend who has been there himself can nip a potential argument with your partner in the bud and help you go back to her – ready to be supportive.

Planning a 'baby moon'

It may seem a long way off yet, but the months before your baby is born are very precious for you as a couple, particularly if this is your first child. This is the last time it will be 'just you two' for quite a while. The next phase, of being pregnant and then giving birth, is going to be one of the most amazing of your lives and a great time to bond with each other over new discoveries. But this means it is even more important to use the time before your child is born to really enjoy each other's company.

During your pregnancy, other family members such as your parents and in-laws may also become more involved in your lives and this can sometimes eclipse you and your partner as a couple, making it doubly important to take time out now. Use this time to touch base and make sure that you are as close as you can be. If you haven't discussed it for a while, make sure the plans you have for your future as a couple still coincide. Any bonds you forge now will only make you stronger as a couple when you face the challenge of becoming parents together.

During this time it has become increasingly common for couples to take a 'baby moon'. A baby moon is a holiday with your partner to relax, spend time together and prepare yourselves for the next step. This is a great idea and it doesn't need to break the bank. A simple weekend away together will serve just as well as a week somewhere exotic. Perhaps leave your laptops and any work worries at home!

Relationships with in-laws, parents, siblings and friends

While bonding with your partner is especially important during your pregnancy, this time can also give you an opportunity to bond with other members of your family, particularly the female members. There's nothing you can share that's quite like exchanging thoughts, feelings and advice on becoming a mother. You may well find that this advice, born out of experience, is invaluable.

However, this is also a sensitive time and, even though the baby isn't born yet, other people's opinions, advice and experiences can sometimes feel overwhelming, or even unwelcome. A little communication, perhaps letting your family know of the type of support and advice you need, can go a long way towards preventing tension at what should be an enjoyable time. This may become even more intense once your baby is born, so it's good to let people know what you want from them at this point.

In-laws

Relationships with in-laws can be tricky at the best of times and a major event like pregnancy can easily awaken latent issues. Emotions can run high and you'll be a victim of pregnancy hormones, so a small disagreement can easily become magnified out of all proportion.

Loyalty

The core of most of the issues that you may have with your in-laws, pregnancy-related or otherwise, stem from questions about where your partner's loyalty lies. Ideally this situation should not arise, but if he had to choose between you and his mother, whose side would he be on? The answer to this, within reason, should be yours. Naturally, he should always maintain a loving relationship with his mother, but as you are now his primary family, it is you he should support. And as the family unit you share with your husband expands with the impending arrival of a new member, this support becomes even more important.

The most common cause of friction with your in-laws during pregnancy is your mother-in-law (or more rarely your father-in-law) being overly vocal about how they think you should be dealing with things. This can vary from offers of unwanted advice, to expressing surprise that you are not doing things the way they did them.

Trying to help

It's important to remember that most of the time advice comes from a good place. Your mother-in-law is simply trying to help by sharing what she has learnt though experience, and is probably quite unaware of how irritating you are finding her suggestions. If you can manage it, just smile and change the subject. If she persists, you could say something like, 'I'm getting so much advice at the moment, it's a bit overwhelming.' She should take the hint. However, if she continues to be overly opinionated, take your partner aside and explain how her behaviour is making you feel. Ask him to have a quiet word with her, as this is less likely to lead to conflict than broaching the subject yourself. Also, knowing that your partner is openly supportive of you goes a long way towards solving the problem itself.

Passing on advice

Another situation you might find yourself in is hearing your mother-in-law's advice being passed on to you by your partner – you might find this irritating. Statements such as, 'Well, my mum thinks this…' or 'My mum says that…' may well make your blood boil. Be aware that he's just trying to help by giving you advice from the most experienced person he knows, but explain that this makes you feel criticised and undermined (he may be completely unaware of the effect this all has on you) and while you appreciate her suggestions, you'd rather ask if you need help. It might also be a good time to tell him that you feel you instinctively know what's best for your unborn baby.

Finally, don't forget that grandparents are going to form an important focus in your child's life. It's likely that not only will grandparent and grandchild share a wonderful bond, but that you will be very grateful for the support they offer as your child grows up.

Your parents and siblings

It's not just in-laws who can be tactless with unwanted advice. Your own mother (and also aunts, sisters or sisters-in-law) may offer 'useful' information and suggestions. Everyone loves to pitch in with advice and experience. But it's important to remember that they love you as a daughter, niece or a sister as much as they love your unborn child and they want to see both of you thrive.

Dealing with your own side of the family can be more straight-forward than dealing with your in-laws, simply because it is usually easier to tell your mother, even light-heartedly, when she is overstepping the mark (although getting her to carry out your wishes may be another matter). Remember that your partner might find your mother's advice just as intrusive as you may find his mother's. Check how he feels about this, and if it is bothering him you could perhaps make sure that at least some of your pregnancy-related conversations with your mother take place when he is out of earshot.

Unique bond

You may find that pregnancy is a time when you can build a unique bond with your own mother. Being about to embark on mother-hood yourself will help you to understand your relationship with her in ways that may have been mystifying before. If you can, take the time to enjoy each other's company and discuss your thoughts and feelings about motherhood and pregnancy. If you don't live near each other, a chat over the phone will serve just as well. Forging bonds now is worth every effort – you will be very grateful for her support once your baby arrives. Don't forget that many of the comments your mother makes are because of her love for you and her excitement about the new grandchild coming into her life.

Your friends

You might already be part of a group of friends who have children, or perhaps you are the first of your friends to become pregnant. Whichever is the case, it's inevitable that your pregnancy will change the relationship you have with your friends in some way.

If some of your friends have children already, they can be a great source of knowledge about child-friendly places in your area. They can also be a great sounding-board if you want to blow off steam. They have been there, done that, and will probably welcome you into the fold of new parenthood with open arms. However, as with siblings or other relations, you might find them offering unwanted advice if they expect you to follow their own parenting choices. Depending on how close you are to the friend in question, you might want to handle this differently, but if you differ in your opinions it's important to show that you are happy with your own parenting choices. Try not to feel pressurised by your friends or enter into any competitiveness about parenting, as this can cause friction in what could be a strong and supportive friendship.

Some of your other friends might be less happy about your pregnancy. They might resent the fact that you're no longer available to go clubbing or able to embark on huge shopping missions with a long liquid lunch in the middle! If this is the case, let them know that your life has changed and perhaps there are other ways for you to have fun. It may be that you lose contact with some of your friends, only to regain it once they themselves become pregnant! This is fine: friendships are always changing and evolving.

Some friends – and you know who they are – are ones with whom you want to share this new phase of your life. For this group, it's important that you talk through any worries you or they might have. Again, sharing your fears can bring you closer together. It's amazing what a little communication can do!

For such a tiny thing, a new baby has a huge impact on the people around him. Bringing a new life into the world is a fantastic opportunity to breathe new life into your relationships and to strengthen the bonds between you, your partner, your families and friends. With good communication, respect and openness, your pregnancy could deepen the warmth and love you feel for those around you.

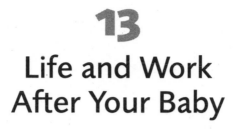

Life and Work After Your Baby

Going Back to Work or Staying at Home?

Apart from starting to think about getting your home ready for the new baby, you also need to think about your own life. One of the first things to consider is what you'd like to do – or, perhaps, what you can afford to do – about work.

If you're in a well-paid, satisfying job and this is your first child, you may want to take your maternity leave and go back to work afterwards. But if your job is not very well paid, not really what you want to do or you just want to spend time being a full-time mum, you might be considering stopping work and staying at home. However, if there is a possibility of going part time in a job you are happy in, perhaps this might be worth exploring. That way you can keep involved in your career, should you wish to return to it more fully later on. Fathers staying at home and becoming the main carer is not the norm at present, but is becoming increasingly popular, so your partner might want to take on the full-time, stay-at-home parenting role while you return to work after maternity leave. Or perhaps you could afford to share the parenting between you and both work part-time, if this can be arranged. It all depends on your individual circumstances and preferences.

Should you take a career break?

Some big employers have their own crèches or are prepared to subsidise your childcare costs. If you're on a low income you might qualify for child tax credits, plus the childcare element, and you can find out about this on the HMRC website (see Resources, page 329). But for most people, the cost of childcare takes a major chunk out of their salary. Once you've done your sums, you might begin to feel that it's simply not worth going back to work, especially if you're expecting twins or are on your second or third pregnancy, as of course the costs of childcare increase with the number of children you have.

You may be one of those mothers who, despite having a fulfilling career, may be able to afford to look after their children full-time and plan to rekindle their work life later on. But it's worth having a hard think about the future and what this would mean for your earning capacity – and your day-to-day satisfaction – in years to come. If you work in a field where a break might mean that it's very difficult to get back into work – because you become out of touch with ever-changing legislation, technology, clients or contacts – you might decide that it's essential to keep working, despite the expense of childcare.

Looking after their own children is so important to some parents that they decide to alter their lifestyles in order to accommodate having one partner at home full-time. This may mean a big drop in joint salary, perhaps more modest holidays, fewer treats, fewer new clothes and only rare trips out, but for you it may be worth the sacrifice.

Maternity Leave and Benefits

It is important to be aware of what you are entitled to when it comes to maternity leave and benefits. Your GP or midwife will be able to give you a basic explanation when you attend your booking appointment (see page 106), but depending on where you work, the amount you receive during maternity leave will vary – some employers are more generous than others.

Once your pregnancy is confirmed and you have told your employer, you will have some additional protection at work and it's a good idea to be clear on what your entitlements are – to ensure that you don't miss out on any of them.

Maternity leave

You can take up to 52 weeks' maternity leave, although this will not all be paid leave (see page 266). The amount of leave you receive doesn't depend on the length of time you have been working for your employer (although your entitlement to maternity pay does).

When you discuss maternity leave with your employer, you need to show them a MATB1 form, which confirms the baby's expected due date. You can get this from your GP or midwife. You must tell your employer that you are pregnant 15 weeks before your due date (this week is called the 'qualifying week' and is used to calculate your statutory benefits), or before that if you can. If you don't realise you are pregnant until after this, you can still get maternity leave – just talk to your employer as soon as you realise you are pregnant.

When should you start your leave?

You, rather than your employer, decides the date you intend to start maternity leave, but you need to give your employer at least 28 days' notice. You can start maternity leave at any time between the beginning of the eleventh week before the baby is due and the week after he is born. If you are off work because of your pregnancy within four weeks of your due date, your employer can decide that your maternity leave starts then, even if you had originally booked it to start later.

If you don't talk to your employer before the eleventh week before your baby is due, they might not agree to the date on which you want your maternity leave to start. If your baby is born prematurely, this is obviously beyond your control and your employer will have to make an exception for you, allowing you to start maternity leave early. If you're an employee, two weeks' maternity leave is compulsory, and you must take four weeks if you work in a factory.

About Statutory Maternity Leave (SML)

Statutory Maternity Leave is divided into two parts: 'ordinary' and 'additional' maternity leave. Ordinary Maternity Leave (OML) is the first 26 weeks of leave. Although you won't get your usual pay, unless your contract allows it, in other respects you are treated as if you are working, so you can still build up holiday entitlement and receive pay rises. You can then take another 26 weeks off, which is called Additional Maternity Leave (AML). AML must run on from OML – you can't go back to work in between.

After you and your employer have agreed when your maternity leave will begin, your employer will have to inform you of your prospective return date within 28 days. They'll probably assume you are taking your full entitlement of 52 weeks.

If you decide to come back before the end of OML you must give 28 days' notice, and if you want to come back to work during AML you have to give at least eight weeks' notice.

Parental leave

All employees with a child under five years old or a disabled child under 18 years of age are entitled to 13 weeks' unpaid parental leave, as long as they've been working for their employer for one year or more. You can take this amount of leave for each child. The statutory maximum you can take at any one time is four weeks (although your employer's parental leave policy might allow you to take more), and you need to give your employer 21 days' notice that you intend to take it. If your employer thinks that this will disrupt business too much, they can ask you to postpone it.

You can take parental leave immediately after maternity leave. So you can extend your SML with parental leave and with any holiday entitlement you have accrued during your maternity leave.

Paternity leave and pay

If your partner is an employee, he may be entitled to up to two weeks' paid paternity leave (this also applies if your partner is a woman). His or her employer might have a more generous paternity leave scheme that would be set out in their contract. If you return to work before the end of your maternity leave your partner might be entitled to take Additional Paternity Leave. See the Directgov website for the latest information: www.direct.gov.uk

Maternity pay

To get Statutory Maternity Pay (SMP), you must have been working for the same employer continuously for at least 26 weeks, into the fifteenth week before your baby is due. It doesn't matter whether you work full- or part-time, but you must have been earning £107 a week or more (for the 2012–13 tax year) to qualify for SMP. If you leave your job after the qualifying week of your pregnancy, you should still get SMP.

If you own a limited company and pay yourself through PAYE, you will get SMP if you meet the conditions.

Many people find that the contractual maternity pay provided by their employer is better than SMP. If it isn't, you can ignore what your contract says and rely on your statutory rights.

You can get SMP for up to 39 weeks. For the first six weeks you get 90 per cent of your average gross weekly pay per week. For the remaining weeks you get the same amount as the first six weeks or £135.45 per week (in 2013), whichever is the lower. If you're taking the full 52 weeks' leave that means the last three months will be unpaid. If you were claiming working tax credit during the paid part of your maternity leave, you can't claim it during the unpaid part.

Maternity Allowance and Employment Support Allowance

If you don't qualify for SMP – because you haven't been working for your employer for long enough, you've changed jobs during your pregnancy or your weekly wage is too low – you might qualify for Maternity Allowance (MA). MA is paid for up to 39 weeks, and is either £135.45 a week (in 2013) or 90 per cent of your weekly earnings, whichever is lower.

If you're registered as self-employed you can't get SMP, but you can usually get MA. You can check the conditions on the DWP website or the Directgov website (see Resources, page 329).

You have to apply for MA through Jobcentre Plus, and you can claim when you're 26 weeks pregnant. Call 0800 055 6688 to get a copy of the form (MA1) or download it from the DWP website. If you can't get MA, you might be able to get employment and support allowance (ESA) for a limited period. The Jobcentre Plus adviser should automatically check whether you can get ESA. If you're unemployed, you may be able to get MA or ESA.

If you are not a permanent resident in the UK, but have a visa that allows you to live and work here, you might still get SMP or MA, it all depends on your employment history. Some visas state you have 'no recourse to public funds', but SMP and MA are not treated as public funds.

Different rules for maternity pay and leave apply to women working in the armed forces or for the police.

Additional support

If you get Income Support or Job Seekers' Allowance, you might qualify for Child Tax Credit, as well as housing benefit and council tax benefit. You could also get vouchers for milk, fruit, vegetables, formula milk and vitamins under the Healthy Start scheme: ask your GP or midwife for an application form, or go to the Healthy Start website (see Resources, page 328).

Sure Start provides maternity grants of £500 (to buy essential baby equipment) for people on these benefits whose baby will be the only child under 16 in the household. If you're expecting twins, triplets or more, and qualify for the Sure Start grant, you get £500 per baby. You can get the application pack from Jobcentre Plus or from the Directgov website at www. direct.gov.uk.

Child benefit

Parents under a certain income threshold will be entitled to child benefit, though legislation is changing at time of writing (2013) and eligibility depends on your income levels. Check your entitlements online or ask your health visitor. If you don't live with your child's other parent, you don't both get the allowance – it will only be paid to one of you. You don't get child benefit automatically – you need to claim, and you can find out how at www. hmrc.gov.uk.

Free prescriptions

Regardless of how much you earn, you are entitled to free prescriptions and dental care during pregnancy and for a year after your baby's birth. You need to fill in the FW8 form, which you can get from your GP, midwife or health visitor; they need to sign it too. If you don't apply before your baby is born, you can still apply afterwards.

To get free dental care, just show your dentist your MATB1 form or your FW8 form while you are pregnant. After you have had your baby, show your FW8, the baby's birth certificate or a 'notification of birth' form, which you can get from your midwife.

Your rights at work

While you are pregnant

You are entitled to work in a safe environment and to take time off for antenatal care appointments (see page 112). The law also protects you from being sacked or demoted for being pregnant or taking maternity leave.

If an employer fails to protect the health and safety of their pregnant workers, it will be automatically considered as sex discrimination. For example, if there is a real risk of violence from others while you are working, you have a right to be given suitable alternative work.

After the baby is born

Your employer should tell you about opportunities for promotion or any relevant job vacancies that come up at your place of work. They should also maintain a 'reasonable' amount of contact with you, to keep you up to date with what is going on at work. You can work up to 10 'keeping in touch' days (this is good for team meetings or training days) during your maternity leave without losing any maternity pay. You are not obliged to work these days and your employer is not obliged to offer them to you.

All women have the right to go back to their old job after the 26 weeks' OML. After the additional 26 weeks of AML, you can go back to your old job if it is reasonably practical. If it isn't, your employer must offer you something with the same rate of pay and terms and conditions.

If you have been in your job for 26 weeks before the qualifying week, your employer must consider your requests for flexible working, or part-time or reduced hours. But considering your request doesn't mean that they have to give you what you've asked for. If they refuse to consider your request, you should talk to the Citizens Advice Bureau (see Resources, page 329) or get legal advice.

Q What if I'm ill when it's time to go back to work?

A You must provide a medical certificate and you should get statutory sick pay (if you normally earn more than £107 a week in 2013). Alternatively your employer might run their own sick pay scheme. If you are not entitled to SSP, you may get ESA. Your employer should tell you how to apply for this.

You are protected by law from unfair dismissal for another four weeks if you become ill at the end of your maternity leave. If you are still ill after this and your employer tries to sack you, it will probably be seen as discrimination. The best people to talk to if this happens would be the staff at your local Citizens Advice Bureau.

Q What if I decide I don't want to go back to my job?

A You must give the notice set out in your contract. You should be paid in lieu for any holiday you haven't taken, including any holiday entitlement built up during your maternity leave. You don't have to repay Statutory Maternity Pay, but your contract might require you to pay back all or part of your Enhanced Maternity Pay (EMP).

If you start working for a different employer while you are still receiving SMP, you must inform your original employer, as you would not be allowed to receive SMP any more.

Q **What if I get pregnant again while I'm still on maternity leave or soon after I return to work?**

A When you are receiving SMP you are entitled to the same benefits as when you are working, so you would have exactly the same rights as on your first maternity leave. You must go back to work, though, even if it is only for a very short time. If your second maternity leave is quite close to your first one, you may not get as much SMP as the first time around. SMP is calculated on your average earnings eight weeks before the qualifying week, so if you were getting maternity pay rather than your full salary at this time, your SMP will be lower the second time around.

Q **I want to carry on breast-feeding when I go back to work – can I?**

A Legally, your employer has to support you if you want to breast-feed at work. You need to tell them in writing that you are breast-feeding and want to continue, and they have to make this possible. Unless your baby is being cared for at a workplace crèche or very close to work, this will probably mean expressing your milk. Your employer needs to give you a break or breaks to do this, a warm and private place to do it (not the toilet) and a fridge in which to store the expressed milk.

Q What if my baby is ill on a day that I am supposed to be at work?

A Your employer should allow you 'reasonable' time off – usually two days or less – to deal with an emergency involving a dependant. This could be, for example, if your nanny falls ill, or your child is too unwell to go to nursery. This time is normally unpaid, unless your contract says otherwise. Some employers will come to amicable agreements with staff, allowing them to take the odd day when their child is ill as 'time off in lieu' (so that you have to make up your hours at another time) or as sick leave. But others will make you take it out of your paid annual leave.

If you are going to have to take more than a couple of days off, you might be able to take it as part of your parental leave (see above), provided that you have been working for your employer for a year or more and haven't already taken your four weeks that year.

If you are refused 'reasonable' time off, are penalised in some way (for example, by not being promoted) or are made redundant because you've taken time off to look after a sick child, you can take your case to an employment tribunal.

Help in your home

Whether you decide to stay at home or intend to go back to work, having a baby is a wonderful experience and heralds a new chapter in your life. However, no one ever said that raising a child is easy! But don't worry: there are options for help for you and your new family. The National Childminding Association (see Resources, page 329) offers guidance on choosing the right childcare options for you.

Maternity nurses

This type of nurse supports you and baby in the weeks, or even months, after the birth and helps you establish a routine at what can be a challenging time. She sleeps in the nursery with the baby and provides bottle-feeds during the night or brings the baby to you for breast-feeds, whichever you prefer. She then changes, comforts and settles the baby afterwards, so that you can go back to sleep. She keeps the baby's room tidy, does his laundry and deals with nappies, and may cook for you, though not for the rest of the family. Maternity nurses are paid upwards of £600 a week, depending on their experience. Good maternity nurses get booked up well in advance, so it's a good idea to plan this as early as you can. Bear in mind that because you engage a maternity nurse to work for you from a certain date, you still have to pay her for that time – even if the baby arrives later than expected. Look online for maternity nurse agencies. Their websites explain exactly what services they offer and provide helpful and informative references from other parents who have used them. Otherwise ask your GP or midwife for recommendations.

Relatives

Unless your relatives live really close by, you are unlikely to be able to rely on your parents or in-laws to help out with childcare. Your mother or mother-in-law may still be in paid work herself, or she may be enjoying such an active retirement that she's reluctant to commit to regular days caring for grandchildren.

However, if a relative can help with looking after your baby, this needs almost as much consideration as employing a professional nanny or child-minder. You might want to pay your relative, so that you don't have to feel beholden to them. Or if they won't accept money, a monthly gift card or treat of some sort could be something to consider. You also have to think about what would happen if your views on childcare differ from theirs: it might be very difficult to challenge your mother-in-law (see also page 255) and far easier to discuss different approaches with a professional nanny or child-minder. If a relative does offer to help you, it's probably a good idea to talk about how they'll care for your baby and what their core beliefs about childcare are, so that anything you strongly disagree with can be discussed and sorted out right at the start.

Mother's help

A mother's help is someone who doesn't live in your home, but who looks after the children and does light housework while you are present in the home. She doesn't necessarily have specific relevant qualifications, although it's a good idea to make sure that she has some first-aid training. The only previous experience she needs is as a babysitter. You may need to pay only the minimum wage (currently £6.08 an hour for over-21s), but if the person taking the job has nanny qualifications, she may command up to £10 an hour.

Au pairs

Au pairs can't look after babies and pre-school children on their own, but they're a great option if you're at home with your children and need an extra pair of hands. You need enough space to give the au pair a home and be able to welcome them as one of the family. They normally work for five hours a day, five days a week, plus two evenings' babysitting. They are not trained in childcare and are usually undertaking the work in order to learn English. You provide their accommodation, food, perhaps organise English classes and pay them £60 a week. You can come to arrangements that involve longer working hours, but you'll need to pay extra.

Nannies

Nannies are an expensive option, but they can be more cost-effective than a day nursery if you've got more than one child. Expect to pay £7 or more an hour, plus tax, national insurance, holiday pay and expenses such as petrol (if they're driving your children around in their own car). Nanny-shares (where you share a nanny with another family, and the children spend some days at your house and some at the other family's house) can provide reassuring continuity of care more affordably, although it's worth bearing in mind that as they get older some babies and small children don't like being moved around between different homes – they prefer being looked after at home in familiar surroundings with their own toys.

Nurseries

Day nurseries can either be stimulating, sociable environments, or overwhelming and confusing for young children – it all depends on the baby's personality and what they are used to. What is certain, though, is that nurseries are pretty expensive and you may well have to pay an enrolment fee and put your baby on a waiting list before they're even born to get a place at a popular one. Nurseries cost from around £500 per month, and up to £1,200 a month in London. Many charge extra if you're late picking up your child, and of course you still have to pay when your child is not well enough to go or when you go away on holiday.

Child-minders

Child-minders are the cheapest and most flexible childcare option, but they will have commitments to older children in their care, such as dropping off and picking up from school, so your baby's day will have to fit around the needs of others, particularly the child-minder's own children. You also have to be prepared for your child to be cared for in the way your child-minder chooses. So, for example, if her children are watching TV, yours will be too. Many child-minders are excellent and provide a 'home-from-home' atmosphere. You can find a list of registered child-minders on your local authority's website. They charge between £3.50 and £5 an hour and you may have to pay extra for meals. Many parents supply their child's nappies, wipes and food.

PART 4

Birth and Beyond

14
Labour and Birth

Throughout the final stages of your pregnancy, you will be focused on the birth. If this is your first pregnancy, you may feel a little anxious about what lies ahead and be concerned about how you will cope. If you have already had a baby, you may be hoping that this time the birth will be different – or that your labour for your second baby will be as straightforward as the first!

Be prepared

It is important to be as prepared for the birth as you can be. Reading up about what may lie ahead can be helpful, but remember that every birth is different and every woman's experience of labour is different too. It is difficult to know how it will affect you as there are so many varying factors that can influence what happens. However, knowing more about what might happen will help you to feel as prepared as you can be.

The last few weeks

You may notice some changes, both physical and emotional, during the final few weeks before your baby arrives. The final stages of pregnancy will be different for each woman, so you may not have all of the following signs or symptoms, but many women experience at least some of these as the birth approaches.

Braxton Hicks contractions

These 'practice' contractions are likely to become more common in the last few weeks of pregnancy. They can occur far earlier in pregnancy and some women experience them on and off for many months, but they tend to be irregular. Although some women find them uncomfortable, they are not usually painful. When you are having a Braxton Hicks contraction your bump will feel hard and tight. (See also page 165.)

As the final weeks or days of pregnancy approach, women often find that their Braxton Hicks contractions become more frequent and more intense. If the contractions start to feel very uncomfortable, changing position and moving around often helps. Some women worry that they have gone into labour if their Braxton Hicks contractions are quite intense, but there are differences since the contractions of labour are regular and become more painful as they go on.

Your baby's position

During the final part of your pregnancy, your baby will get into position in preparation for the birth, a process known as 'engagement'. The baby's head will drop down into your pelvis and you will usually be aware of a change of position. Once his head is engaged, you may find that you walk in a different way and that the pressure on your bladder means that you need to go to the loo more frequently. Engagement can happen at any time during the final stages of pregnancy, but it is usually earlier for first-time mothers and can occur at any time from about 36 weeks onwards. However, some babies don't drop down until the last minute, when labour begins.

Posterior position

Sometimes, babies don't get into the best position for labour. They may be in a posterior position, with their backs towards their mother's backs rather than their fronts (which is the easiest way for them to be born). Labour can be more painful if your baby is in a posterior position, but most babies turn around to the anterior position in labour if there are good contractions.

Breech position

If your baby has his bottom rather than his head downwards, this is known as being in a 'breech' position (see also page 204). Try not to worry if your baby is in this position in the last few weeks, as most breech babies move into a better position before the birth; only 4 per cent, at most, are still in this position by the time they are due. If your baby remains in a breech position, the team looking after you will discuss the options.

The show

You may have a discharge, known as the 'show', before labour starts. This happens when the plug of mucus (which may be streaked with blood and a brownish or pinkish colour), which has been keeping the cervix closed off during pregnancy, is now released. Sometimes this only happens once you are actually in labour, but you may find it happens a few days beforehand.

Induction

If your pregnancy goes well, it is quite common for it to go on past your due date. This is not an issue until you are two weeks late, when there can be a higher risk of problems with the baby's growth.

Sometimes it is difficult to calculate exactly when your due date is, especially if your periods are irregular, if you had been using hormonal contraception or had been breast-feeding. An early scan is often helpful in dating your pregnancy accurately and ensuring that it doesn't go on for too much longer.

If doctors have concerns that your pregnancy risks becoming too prolonged, or are worried about your health or your baby's health, you may find that you need to have your labour induced. Other reasons for induction may include diabetes (see page 193), high blood pressure (see page 191), ruptured membranes, or problems with your baby such as him being unusually small or large. There are a number of different methods that may be used to start labour, and often more than one of these will be used at the same time.

Membrane sweeping

If your baby is late or you are towards the last two weeks of your pregnancy, your doctor or midwife may offer to do a membrane sweep before considering other induction methods. This can reduce the risk of your baby being very overdue. It is an internal examination, during which the doctor or midwife massages, or 'sweeps', around the cervix. The aim is to separate the membranes of the sac containing your baby from the womb, as this can release hormones that help to stimulate labour. Having a sweep can be quite uncomfortable and there can be some spotting afterwards plus period-like pains. If the membrane sweep doesn't induce labour first time around, your doctor or midwife may offer to try again before you consider induction.

Artificial rupture of membranes

If your cervix is already dilated, doctors may suggest breaking your waters, which is known as 'artificial rupture of membranes'. A small instrument is used to pierce the membranes and break the waters. This doesn't hurt and once the waters have broken, your contractions may begin. If not, contractions will be stimulated with an intravenous drug called syntocinon (see overleaf). This is started at a low dose at first, building up the strength and regularity of the contractions. You will be monitored when you are on this drug to check the contractions and to make sure that your baby is doing well.

Induction of labour

The most common method of induction is to give prostaglandins. These are naturally released in labour and a synthetic version is given to you to help bring on contractions. It may be given as a controlled-release vaginal pessary, a vaginal gel or tablet. You will be monitored before and after it is given. It can take a while for it to take effect and a second dose may sometimes be necessary. If your waters don't break, this may need to be done artificially and a syntocinon drip (see below) may be needed if your contractions are not strong or regular.

In some birthing units, you will be allowed to go home between doses of prostaglandins, as long as your waters haven't broken and you are not in labour.

If you have had a Caesarean section before, you will need to talk to your doctor about whether you will be suitable for induction if you choose to try for a vaginal delivery. Generally, you would be monitored in hospital all the time if prostaglandins were used and the doses given would be lower. Some hospitals prefer to use a small balloon introduced into the cervix to help open it rather than use drugs if you have had a previous Caesarean section.

Occasionally, in about 5 per cent of cases, prostaglandins can overstimulate the womb and if this happens you will be given another drug to counteract the contractions.

Syntocinon

Once your waters have broken, either on their own or by artificial rupture of the membranes, if the contractions do not start the doctors may suggest syntocinon to bring on the contractions. This drug has to be administered intravenously, so a drip will be set up so that it goes directly into your bloodstream. Syntocinon usually brings on quite strong contractions fairly quickly, and they can be painful, so you may need additional pain relief. You will also have to be monitored continuously to check that these strong contractions aren't causing your baby any distress.

'Natural' methods of bringing on labour

If your baby is overdue, you are likely to hear all kinds of old wives' tales about different ways to bring on labour, and people may suggest anything from taking long walks and drinking raspberry leaf tea to eating curry and pineapples. Acupuncture, castor oil, homeopathic drugs and sexual intercourse (though not after your waters have broken) may also be suggested. Many people swear by one idea or another because babies have arrived after they've tried them. However, this may be just coincidence, since babies tend to come along when they are ready to and there is no clinical evidence that any of these methods are effective. Nipple stimulation, however, may be of some benefit since it releases the hormone oxytocin, which stimulates uterine contractions.

Pain relief and induction

If this is your first labour and you're planning not to have any pain relief at all, it's still a good idea to find out about it, just in case, because you might change your mind when labour gets under way. Labour doesn't always go to plan or your reactions to pain might be different to what you expect, so you need to know about all the options.

If your labour has to be induced, it is often more painful and longer than a spontaneous labour might be. For this reason, you may need to reconsider the decisions you made in your birth plan (see page 129) if you'd hoped to be able to give birth with minimal pain relief. Take advice from your midwife when deciding on the best course of action.

Being relaxed and calm

Labour is usually painful at some level and the calming words 'relax' and 'give birth' might not sound realistic. It's normal to feel a certain amount of anxiety about the big day, but the more relaxed you are during labour, the better it's likely to go. During labour you naturally produce oxytocin and endorphins (both of which have 'feel-good' effects), and if you're relaxed, you produce more of these. Feeling calm and controlled during labour will help you to feel less stressed and tired, and will give you the energy to cope with contractions and with pushing your baby out at the end. A supportive birth partner, whether this is your partner, a doula or your midwife, can help you feel calmer and have a very positive effect on the way you perceive birth and, as a consequence, the way the birth goes.

Massage

Massage can be very helpful for pain relief in labour and your partner may be able to massage you – it is an excellent way of involving him in the birth. You may want to use essential oils, but you should check with a qualified aromatherapist first since some oils may not be suitable for use during pregnancy and birth.

Aromatherapy oils

If you are giving birth at home, some aromatherapy oils may be helpful and you can use an oil burner to diffuse them. If you are giving birth in hospital, you may not be able to do this, but you can still use the oils in a compress. If you are interested in using aromatherapy oils in labour, talk to an aromatherapist about how best to do this and which oils to use.

Homeopathic remedies

Homeopathic remedies are popular for pain relief in labour, but you must consult a professional homeopath rather than just selecting what you think might be appropriate yourself. They will recommend the different remedies you may want to use at different stages of labour. Ask whether he or she can provide you with a homeopathic birthing kit containing the correct remedies. Some midwives and doctors will be more supportive of the idea of homeopathic remedies than others, which you may want to bear in mind.

The impact of yoga on the birth

Yoga classes are very popular during pregnancy, but it is very important that you make sure the class is specifically for yoga in pregnancy as normal yoga is not always suitable and could even be dangerous. Many yoga teachers will include tips for relaxation during the birth itself. These may include helpful positions and breathing and visualisation techniques. These can be very beneficial when you go into labour as they can help you approach the event feeling calmer and more relaxed, and enable you to deal with pain more effectively. (See also page 97.)

Water birth

Going through labour and possibly giving birth in water is a good idea because water can be so soothing and give you a feeling of weightlessness. Lying in warm water can help support you and can relieve the pain of contractions. If you are in the early stages of labour, you may want to ask if you can have a bath, though this is something that it is best to discuss with your midwife well in advance as it needs to be planned for. You may choose to spend labour in water, for pain relief, and then get out of the pool when it comes to actually giving birth. Or you may want to give birth in the water too. Some hospitals and birthing centres have pools, but this may not always be an option.

If your pregnancy and labour so far have been straightforward, water births are a good form of pain relief, but you may be advised against this method if there are any complications such as foetal distress. It is important that you can still be monitored safely and that your baby can be delivered easily by the midwife. Therefore your GP or midwife may suggest that you remain in the water for pain relief, but not for the birth itself.

Self-hypnosis

Some women try self-hypnosis techniques, which are often taught in hypno-birthing or in active birth methods, where you can move around during the birth. If you are interested in these, you may want to find out whether there are any classes or practitioners in your area. An online search will point you in the right direction.

Gas and air (Entonox)

You control the gas and air yourself by taking as many breaths of it as you like and it leaves your body within minutes of you stopping breathing it. It takes 30 seconds to take effect, so it's important to start breathing it as soon as you feel a contraction coming on. You can use Entonox while you're in the water during a water birth.

The gas in gas and air is nitrous oxide (laughing gas) and it can cause you to feel light-headed or even sick, making it difficult to concentrate on your contractions, so you may need help from your midwife in using it. You might have to stop using it once you get towards the end of your labour. Its painkilling effects are fairly mild.

TENS machine

Transcutaneous Electrical Nerve Stimulation (TENS) machines use tiny electrical impulses to intervene with the way your brain receives pain signals during labour, so your pain can seem reduced. The impulses also stimulate your body to release endorphins, which are natural painkillers. You can use a TENS machine in early labour and at the same time as you're using Entonox (gas and air).

If you're giving birth in hospital, check whether the hospital has TENS machines available. Even if it does, you might find that there isn't one free right when you need it, so you might prefer to hire or even buy one, as you can acquire them for less than £40 and you can buy 'mini' versions for even less. You can't use them in birthing pools as they are electronic. There are no side-effects. A point to consider is that there is no evidence to show that TENS machines are an effective method of pain relief and some women don't feel they do much for them and may even find them irritating.

Pethidine

Pethidine is an injected opiate drug, similar to morphine. You can be given it during the first stage of labour, before you start to push. If you are near to pushing, you cannot be given pethidine because it affects the baby, so the midwife or doctor will check how dilated you are before they administer it. Pethidine can take up to 20 minutes to work and will then be topped up every two or three hours.

The advantages of pethidine are that it reduces pain and relaxes you. It can make the earlier stages of labour easier to cope with and can delay or even prevent you having to progress to an epidural. If you're going through a very long labour, pethidine can give you the chance to sleep for a little while. Midwives are able to give pethidine, even at home births, meaning that you don't need to wait for a doctor to do it.

Unfortunately pethidine does have quite a few disadvantages, including making you drowsy or dizzy. It makes some women feel sick and even vomit. For this reason, it is usually given with an anti-sickness drug, but even that might not prevent you from being sick. Some women report that pethidine made them feel out of control, and, occasionally, that it didn't have much effect on their pain. If you are planning a water birth, you can't be given pethidine less than two hours before you go into the birthing pool.

Pethidine won't be given if you are close to giving birth because it can cross the placenta and it may make your baby drowsy and affect his breathing. It can also interfere with his sucking reflex, so it might take you longer to establish breast-feeding.

Some hospitals offer diamorphine or meptazinol (Meptid) as an alternative to pethidine. These are administered via an injection to the thigh or intravenously. They have similar disadvantages to pethidine in that they can make you sleepy and/or nauseous and can affect your baby. Anecdotal and some research evidence seems to show that they're better at relieving pain than pethidine, and that the negative effects on the baby are reduced. However,

Meptid is so much more expensive than the other two that you might not even be offered it.

Even after having one of these drugs, some women find that they can't cope with their pain. This means they might be offered an epidural.

Epidural

An epidural is an injection into the epidural space in your spine. It reduces feeling to the lower part of your body and is usually given when you're partially dilated and the contractions are intense.

Epidurals can only be given in hospital because they can only be administered by an anaesthetist. Most labour wards have anaesthetists on call at all times, but sometimes they get busy and there may be a wait for one to attend you.

Epidurals can be used from early on in labour and are useful if it is likely that your labour will turn out to be long or difficult. They block the pain that you feel from the contractions and also pain in the vaginal area. You will be given a local anaesthetic first and a thin tube is inserted into the space around the nerves of the spinal cord in the lower part of your back so that more anaesthetic can be injected later. This can be an uncomfortable process, but once the epidural is in and working, the pain relief is very effective. Your anaesthetist will talk you through the procedure and the possible side-effects before giving the epidural to you.

The main advantage of an epidural is that most women find that the reduced sensation of pain means you can cope with the labour better if it's expected to go on for several more hours. The disadvantage is that the labour may slow down, so you may need to take syntocinon (see page 284) to speed the labour up again. In addition, you're more likely to have a ventouse or forceps (see pages 303 and 302) delivery than if you don't have an epidural. You will be less mobile with an epidural and need to be continuously monitored in labour. However, these disadvantages might be outweighed by the comfort of the pain relief.

The most common side-effect of an epidural is low blood pressure and this risk is usually reduced by giving extra intravenous fluid before you have it. Other side-effects include itchy skin, shivering and nausea, and around 12.5 per cent of women find that (for a number of reasons) the pain-reducing effect of an epidural doesn't work. Serious complications are rare. You still have some feeling in your legs and feet and can probably move around on the bed a little.

If you're having a planned Caesarean, you're more likely to have a spinal anaesthetic, which employs a similar technique, though the anaesthetic is injected directly into the spinal fluid to give more rapid and effective pain relief. It cannot be topped up like an epidural, so it will wear off after a time. The pain block will temporarily paralyse your legs, so you won't be able to move them. It is not suitable for use during early labour as it does not last as long and cannot be topped up in the same way as an epidural. If your Caesarean section is under epidural or spinal anaesthetic, you will be awake and your partner can be with you.

Local anaesthetic

Unless you've already had one, you'll be given a small injection of local anaesthetic if you have to have an episiotomy (see also page 304). This acts very quickly and doesn't interfere with your contractions. An episiotomy is a cut to the perineum (between the vagina and anus), and is given – usually in an emergency – to avoid a major tear or to allow the baby to be helped out during the birth. Minor tears, which may or may not need stitching, heal more quickly than episiotomies.

General anaesthetic

It is no longer common to give a general anaesthetic for labour and birth. However, it may be considered if you are unable to have an epidural or a spinal anaesthetic, or if these have been tried and have been unsuccessful and the baby needs to be delivered immediately. If you are having an elective Caesarean section (see page 306) you will be asked not to eat for four to six hours before surgery, since if you have eaten there's a risk that it could cause problems if you were to be sick. If you had an emergency Caesarean and needed a general anaesthetic, a drug would be given to neutralise the acid contents of your stomach to reduce this risk. If you have a general anaesthetic, your partner will not be able to be in the theatre when your baby is born. You will feel drowsy for some time afterwards, until the drugs wear off.

The first stage of labour

Labour is divided into three different stages. Women often worry about knowing when labour has started, and it is quite common for people to go rushing off to hospital thinking that their baby is on the way, only to be sent home again because what they are actually experiencing is just Braxton Hicks contractions (see page 165).

Contractions

The contractions of labour are different from Braxton Hicks contractions and they are often the first sign of labour. While

Braxton Hicks contractions are irregular and don't usually hurt, labour contractions become increasingly regular and increasingly intense and painful. If you change position or move around, Braxton Hicks contractions will usually fade away, but the contractions of labour are not affected by this and will persist. You will be encouraged to be mobile in early labour as this helps the contractions and dilation as gravity helps the baby's head push on the cervix.

Before the event you may wonder what contractions actually feel like, and the reality is that they are probably different for each person. There is usually a period-type pain across the lower part of your abdomen, but there may also be backache and leg pains too. It is quite common to experience diarrhoea in the early stages of labour.

Initially, there will be quite long gaps between contractions, but as your labour becomes more established, the contractions become closer together and more painful. Sometimes you will find that you have a very strong contraction followed by a weaker one and this is perfectly normal.

The waters breaking

Your waters will usually break at some point during labour. This can happen before the contractions start, but it most often occurs during the first stage of labour. Sometimes your midwife will have to break the waters for you (see page 283) – most often to speed labour along. Try to time your contractions so that you know how far apart they are. Perhaps this is something your partner could help with as you may find it too hard to concentrate and keep track. The contractions help with dilation and shortening of your cervix as it opens to let the baby out.

Gradual opening

During labour the cervix thins as it gradually opens and the midwife or doctor can check how your labour is progressing by seeing how dilated the cervix is. They measure this in centimetres. This process can take many hours.

The latent stage of labour

Initially, the early part of labour is known as the 'latent stage' and this can take many hours, or even days and weeks. During this phase the cervix begins to open, soften and shorten. The contractions, though uncomfortable, will not be as intense and regular as when the first stage of labour begins.

First stage

'Established' or 'active' labour is from when the cervix is 4 cm (1½ in) dilated until it is fully dilated. The amount of time the cervix takes to dilate varies hugely from one person to another and it is usually longer in a first pregnancy, when it can take around 12 hours.

The last phase of the first stage of labour is usually the most intense phase because the cervix finally opens fully. You may find that you feel quite different during this phase; you may be irritable, shaky or shivery. Or you may be sick or at least feel nauseous. At this point you may feel that you can't carry on and you may even feel a little weepy. The inability to feel comfortable or to relax between contractions may seem unbearable. You may have been dealing with labour very well up until this point, but suddenly start wanting more pain relief.

The second stage – delivery

Once the cervix is fully dilated, you are in the final stages before your baby is born. In the initial (passive) phase, there is no pushing and the contractions help to bring the baby's head down further into the vagina, and then the active phase begins, when you push the baby out.

Bearing down
Once it is time to push, your midwife will help you to get into the most comfortable position and will teach you how to 'bear down' as long as possible during contractions – to help you to push the baby out. As the contraction occurs, she will ask you to hold your breath and bear down. This may happen every two or three minutes and you may need to take several breaths during the contraction, which may last between 60 and 90 seconds. It is important to listen to your midwife so that you can time your pushing with the contractions. Work with your midwife to get the most out of pushing with each contraction. You will probably feel a strong urge to push when each contraction arrives and you can then catch your breath with deep breathing in between contractions.

Birthing positions
There are a number of different positions for giving birth and you may want to squat, be on all-fours, stand up or lie down. If your partner wants to assist you, perhaps he can help support you – if you want to squat, for example.

Crowning
As the baby's head comes down, it can be seen through the vagina and you may be encouraged to feel it yourself. At first, it

slips back in after each contraction, but gradually more appears ('crowning') and your midwife will apply some pressure to the perineum to ensure that the baby's head doesn't come out too quickly, reducing the risk of tearing. You will feel a stinging sensation and you may be asked to stop pushing at that point so that your perineum can stretch safely and thin out as much as possible, to make delivery easier. Sometimes it is necessary to make a small cut in the perineum on the lower right side (an episiotomy) to prevent you from tearing excessively.

The birth

Once the baby's head appears, the midwife checks his neck to ensure that the cord isn't wrapped around it and then the shoulders appear. The rest of the baby's body then slips out easily. If the baby is fine and there have been no problems in labour, the baby will be given to you so that you can hold him straight away. This is an important part of the bonding process and you will be encouraged to hold him 'skin to skin'. If you are not able to do this for any reason your partner can do it instead of you. Even if the baby needs to be seen by the doctors first, as soon as they are satisfied with his condition he will be brought back so that you can hold him.

Cutting the cord

Once the baby is delivered and his cord has stopped pulsing, it will be clamped and then cut (your partner may be asked whether he wants to do this). You can hold your baby while this is being done.

Post-birth tests

The midwife then checks that the baby is healthy and he will be given an Apgar score. This score awards points out of 10 for his heart rate, breathing, skin colour, reflexes and movement. It is done at one minute after birth and then at five minutes and assesses whether the baby needs medical attention. A score of seven or above is considered normal. Even if the score is low initially, in the majority of cases the baby will be fine. He will be given a general examination to make sure that he is generally healthy and he will be weighed and measured too.

Breast-feeding

It is good to try to breast-feed your baby as soon as possible after birth, as this helps your womb to contract and it decreases bleeding. It is important to do this, even if you do not intend to breast-feed your baby in the long-term. Sometimes, if there are any signs of distress, or if the baby is premature, he may need to be assessed by

Progress during labour

During a normal labour, the cervix dilates from 0–10 cm and the baby's head descends into the pelvis and through the vagina. The baby's head is an oval shape and the contractions have to be strong and frequent to help the baby out. His head needs to be flexed, or bent, towards his chest, in order for the smallest part to pass through the pelvis first. As his head comes into contact with the mother's pelvic floor, it rotates and the head extends for the delivery itself.

If the back of your baby's head faces the wrong way, either towards your back or more towards one side than the other, this makes it more difficult for him to be born. You may be asked to change your position to help the baby rotate, or you may need help with the delivery.

a paediatrician first to ensure that there are no concerns. Your baby will be handed back to you as soon as possible.

The third stage of labour

For a short while after your baby has been born, your contractions will usually stop and the placenta will be delivered about 15 minutes later. Usually you will be given an injection as soon as the baby is born to help the placenta to be expelled efficiently. This reduces any risk of haemorrhage. The team looking after you will need to check it carefully to make sure that it is all present and that nothing has been left inside you. You will be checked for any tears that need stitching, which will be done straight away.

Monitoring in labour

Your progress during labour is charted on a record sheet called a 'partogram', which is kept safely with your notes. This is filled in from when your labour is established and it records how your cervix dilates during labour. It allows those looking after you to see whether your labour is slower than average and whether you may need some intervention such as the waters being broken or syntocinon being given (see page 284).

Your baby's heartbeat will be monitored during labour to help detect any signs that he is distressed or is short of oxygen. Although it is quite common for there to be some changes in your baby's heart rate, it is very uncommon for a baby to suffer from lack of oxygen.

During your antenatal care, you will be categorised as being at 'high' or 'low' risk during labour and your monitoring will be tailored accordingly. There are various methods used to monitor your baby's heartbeat – an ear piece called the Pinnart, which the midwife can place on your abdomen and listen for the heartbeat, a hand-held Doppler ultrasound (sonicaid) and an electronic foetal monitor called a cardiotocogram (CTG).

Intermittent monitoring

If you have a low-risk labour and no problems occur, your baby will be monitored intermittently. You will be monitored once every 15 minutes in the first stage and then after every contraction in the second stage.

Continuous monitoring

If there are abnormalities of the baby's heart rate or there are risk factors (such as a small baby, diabetes or high blood pressure) your baby's heartbeat will be monitored continuously using a cardiotocogram (CTG). You will be attached to the monitor by straps around your abdomen. This also picks up the frequency and duration of your contractions. The baby's heartbeat can be checked with a monitor placed on the abdomen or by using one attached to his head via a small clip.

There is no benefit in continuous monitoring if your pregnancy is low-risk and evidence shows that this leads to an unnecessary rate of medical interventions. Also, being on the CTG restricts how mobile you can be in labour and affects the positions you may wish to adopt.

Sometimes the CTG will show abnormalities and if they persist and are of concern, a small sample of blood can be taken from the baby's head. This is done using a small instrument, which is passed through your vagina so that the baby's head can be seen, and then a spot of blood is drawn into a tube. This gives a much more accurate assessment of the baby's well-being. However, this should not be done if the baby shows severe signs of distress, has bleeding problems or if you have an infection that can be transmitted, such as HIV or hepatitis.

Difficulties during labour

Although labour often follows a fairly straightforward pattern, there are some common problems that can arise that may make it slower or more difficult to deal with.

Posterior labour

If the baby is lying with the back of his head against your spine, he is not in the ideal position for birth. It can cause what is sometimes called a 'backache labour' because you experience lower back pain. It can also prolong labour because the angle of the baby's head won't be ideal. Usually babies gradually move into a better position during labour, but sometimes they may need help to be born with forceps or a ventouse delivery (see overleaf).

A long labour

First babies often take longer to be born, but sometimes labour can go on for too long, with weak contractions and the cervix dilating only very slowly. If the labour is slow, or the baby's heart rate is abnormal, your medical team may try to speed things up by breaking your waters with artificial rupture of membranes (see page 283). This stimulates contractions and gives a picture of the amniotic fluid. If the fluid is clear, this is reassuring, but if it is stained with meconium (see page 173), meaning that the baby has opened his bowel, this can be a sign of foetal distress.

You may be given syntocinon (see also page 284), a synthetic form of the natural hormone oxytocin, which stimulates contractions, if your labour is going slowly, the contractions have become less frequent and the cervix is not dilating. Good contractions are essential, not only for the cervix to dilate but also for the baby to descend into the pelvis and his head to rotate. If your waters haven't already broken, this will be done artificially before you are given syntocinon to see if it speeds up the labour. If it doesn't, you will be given a drip with syntocinon. You will be monitored continuously to ensure your baby is fine and that the contractions are not too strong.

Forceps or ventouse delivery

Sometimes help is needed to enable your baby to be born if he is distressed or if you aren't able to push him out because your contractions are not strong enough or his position makes it more difficult. In this case either forceps or ventouse delivery may be considered.

Forceps

Forceps are like big tongs, which are inserted into your vagina to fit around your baby's head. Gentle pulling on the forceps to coincide with the contractions helps the baby's head to come out.

Ventouse

The ventouse is a plastic or metal suction cup that is applied to the baby's head. Suction pressure is applied, and the baby's head is delivered with the contractions. The ventouse helps the baby's head to rotate and it corrects his overall position in order to ease delivery.

Decision and preparation

Both forceps and ventouse deliveries are only performed by a qualified doctor, and can only be carried out if the baby's head is low in the pelvis. A ventouse delivery is not suitable if the baby is less than 34 weeks.

The doctor will make sure that you have satisfactory pain relief before either of these types of delivery takes place and if you do not have an epidural in place you will be given an injection of local anaesthetic. The choice of which instrument to use depends mainly on the individual preference of the doctor, although a ventouse is better if the baby needs to be rotated and is often a first choice as it is less likely to cause any problems to your vagina or back passage.

The forceps and ventouse can be very successful at helping you to have a vaginal delivery. The ventouse can leave a temporary swelling on the baby's head from the suction, but this usually goes after a few days. The forceps can leave small marks on either side of the baby's face, but these also disappear after a few days. It is rare for ventouse or forceps to cause any risks to the baby, as a Caesarean section (see page 306) is usually done after a few pulls if the baby hasn't been born.

Episiotomy and tearing

If the baby is having difficulty being born, your doctor or midwife may decide to make a small cut in your perineum to help him out. This procedure is known as an 'episiotomy' and it may be given if the baby is stuck or seems distressed. You will be given a local anaesthetic if an episiotomy is necessary. If you have an episiotomy you will have stitches afterwards and these can be uncomfortable for a while, but they usually heal up within a month. About one in seven women in the UK have an episiotomy during labour.

During vaginal delivery the perineum may tear when the baby's head comes out and this occurs in about 85 per cent of all cases. If you have a small tear, known as a 'first-degree' tear, this may be left to heal naturally. A deeper tear, 'second-degree' or 'third-degree' tear, will need stitching.

If you need stitches

Once you have had your baby, your midwife or doctor will check the extent of the tear and episiotomy to see whether you need stitches. If you do, you will be given some local anaesthetic and when the area is numb, the perineum will be stitched. These stitches are dissolvable and so do not require removal. Occasionally the tear can be more extensive and involve the anal sphincter (third-degree tear) or rectum (fourth-degree tear). You will need to be taken into theatre and a spinal or epidural inserted, if one is not in place already. The anal sphincter muscles will need to be repaired and antibiotics and laxatives given to you to ensure you do not strain on the stitches. If you have a third- or fourth-degree tear you should be reviewed by a doctor in a specialised clinic to ensure that the muscles have healed and you have no problems with bowel control.

Cord prolapse

This happens when the membranes break and the cord is below the baby's head. This is more likely if the baby is not head down and the head has not become engaged, with multiple pregnancies, and when there is excessive fluid around the baby. There is a danger that the cord could go into spasm and become compressed, which would reduce the blood supply to the baby, so an emergency Caesarean section (see overleaf) should be performed immediately.

Shoulder dystocia

This is when there is difficulty in delivering the baby's shoulders after his head has emerged. It is more likely to occur with large babies, but it can be hard to predict. If there is difficulty in delivering the baby, the medical staff will perform some manoeuvres to help guide his shoulders out. This involves you placing your thighs up onto your abdomen, while a doctor presses on the top of the pubic bone, rotating the baby from within to deliver the shoulder and performing an episiotomy. As this can be a difficult delivery, a paediatrician will be present to check that your baby is all right.

Postpartum haemorrhage

This is a medical emergency and early diagnosis and administration of blood are essential. It is common to lose some blood after the birth of your baby, but having a haemorrhage, or excessive bleeding, is rare. The commonest reason for this happening is that the uterus does not contract after delivery. Other causes include trauma to the vagina or cervix and a retained placenta. A drip will be inserted to give you fluids and drugs to contract the uterus, which will be rubbed to stimulate a contraction. The vagina and cervix will then be examined to ensure that there is no bleeding from a tear. The doctor will examine the womb and pressure can be applied by the insertion of a balloon inside it. Very occasionally, if the bleeding does not stop you will need other procedures to help stop it, which include compression stitches around the womb, the injection of a gel into the vessels to block the blood supply to the womb and, very occasionally, a hysterectomy. Over the past decade the management of postpartum haemorrhage has really improved and the risk of hysterectomy has declined as well.

Caesarean section

Some women prefer the idea of having a Caesarean section to a vaginal delivery, but normally a Caesarean will only be considered if there is a specific reason why giving birth naturally would not be in the best interests of either you or your baby. Reasons for having a Caesarean section may include:

- The baby becomes very distressed in labour.

- Twin pregnancy.

- Very small birth canal or the baby's head being too large to fit through the pelvis.

- Severe pre-eclampsia (see page 191).

● Viral infections such as HIV.

● Placenta praevia (a condition where the placenta covers part of the entrance to the womb).

● Baby in a breech position (see page 204).

● Medical conditions that might make normal delivery risky.

For most women, a vaginal birth is preferable, but if there are specific reasons for a Caesarean, your doctor or midwife will discuss this with you. More and more women are having Caesarean sections now, but if you have had one in the past this doesn't automatically mean that it will be the best option for you again, so it is important to talk this through with your doctor. The majority of mothers who opt for a vaginal delivery after having had a previous Caesarean section are successful in giving birth vaginally. If you have had more than one Caesarean, you may be advised that you will need to have any future babies by Caesarean section. There is a very small risk of the scar coming apart ('scar dehiscence') (1 per cent) and you will be monitored carefully during your labour for this. If you are aiming to have a vaginal delivery, you may be asked to have your baby in hospital, where you will be closely monitored.

Some women will have an elective Caesarean, where the decision has been made before labour starts, and it is now possible to request to have one even if there are no medical reasons to make it necessary. Caesareans are such a common procedure that there can be a tendency to forget that this is a major operation. However, you should be aware that there are higher risks associated with having a Caesarean, such as wound infection, longer recovery time, deep-vein thrombosis, pulmonary embolism and postpartum haemorrhage. You may also find that it takes longer to recover after a Caesarean delivery than a vaginal birth; this is important to remember as you will need to be quite mobile to look after your new baby. In addition, it can take longer for the baby to adjust after the birth, since being born the 'normal' way is part of his preparation for life outside the womb. It may take more time to establish breast-feeding after a Caesarean too.

An emergency Caesarean may be needed if labour doesn't progress as anticipated or if the baby becomes distressed. This can be difficult if you have been hoping for a natural birth, but it is important to try not to feel disappointed as a decision to go ahead with a Caesarean is undertaken in the interests of your health and your baby's.

The Caesarean operation is carried out by a doctor, usually under epidural or spinal anaesthetic rather than general anaesthetic. This makes it safer and allows you to be awake and have your partner with you. You may both be screened off at the head end so that you do not need to see what is going on. A small incision is made in the lower abdomen along the bikini line. The baby is lifted out, the placenta is removed and then the wound is stitched. The screen can be removed when the baby comes out so that you can see him 'being born'.

Pre-term labour

If you go into labour before you are 37 weeks pregnant, it is considered a 'pre-term' labour and it happens to about one baby in thirteen. There isn't always a reason why a baby is born early, but you may be more at risk if any of the following apply to you:

- If you've had a premature baby before.

- If you've had a late miscarriage before.

- If you are expecting more than one baby.

- If you've had surgery on your cervix.

- If you've had a late termination of pregnancy in the past.

- If you use recreational drugs.

- If you've suffered from collagen and autoimmune diseases.

- If you have had recurrent urinary tract infections.

The first thing you may notice is the start of painful contractions, but in about one-third of cases, pre-term labour begins with the waters breaking (see page 294). If either of these takes place, you should contact your hospital so that you can be assessed. You will be examined and you may have an internal examination to check whether your cervix is dilating and the waters have broken. You may notice a watery vaginal discharge. A swab will be taken to check for fibronectin, a substance produced by the foetal membranes. If this test is positive, you are at higher risk of progressing in labour. You will also be tested for any preliminary signs of infection, usually with a urine test, blood tests and a vaginal swab. The baby will be also be monitored.

It is quite common for women not to go into labour and to remain under observation. If you are under 36 weeks pregnant and in labour you will be given a drug to try to stop the contractions and allow time to give you steroids, which help mature the baby's lungs. Breathing problems are very common in premature babies.

If your waters have broken, you will be observed for any sign of infection by monitoring your temperature and doing blood tests. If there is any sign of infection, your baby may need to be born sooner rather than later. Infection is thought to be the cause of many cases of pre-term labour where the waters break. If everything looks fine, you won't need to stay in hospital, but will be monitored with blood tests twice a week and you will be shown how to check your temperature and look for signs of infection. You may be given antibiotics as they can reduce risks for both you and your baby. It may be suggested that you should be induced once you get past 34 weeks – to reduce the risk of infection.

If there is a risk that your baby will be born before 37 weeks, it is important that you give birth in a unit that has the right facilities and expertise to care for your pre-term baby. If your baby is born very early, the level of expertise needed will be higher. Although care for pre-term babies has improved greatly, babies who are born before 28 weeks are at greater risk as their lungs and major organs are not yet fully mature.

If you have had a previous pre-term delivery or a late miscarriage, a cervical-length scan may be done as a shorter cervical length is related to a high risk of pre-term delivery. You may be offered a cervical stitch, although there is some controversy about how effective this may be.

Changing your birth plan

Sometimes women are upset if their birth hasn't gone exactly as anticipated when they compiled the birth plan (see page 128). However, labour can be unpredictable, so it is important to keep an open mind in order to avoid disappointment. The outcome everyone aims for is that both you and your baby are safe, with no long-term consequences.

There is always a possibility that you may need a Caesarean section and about 25 per cent of all babies are born by Caesarean (see page 306). The risk of having a Caesarean is higher if this is your first baby and much lower if you have had a previous vaginal delivery. It is a good idea to be aware of this risk, especially if this is your first pregnancy, when labour and delivery are often slower and more complicated.

For first-time mothers who opt to deliver at home or in birthing centres, it is quite common to have to transfer to a hospital during labour and this can happen in as many as 20 per cent of births. If you have set your heart on a different sort of birth this may not be ideal, but it is important that you get the right care at the right time in the right place.

For the Birth Partner: Your Role During the Birth

Knowing how best to help and support your partner during labour isn't always easy. Labour may not be as you'd expected it, and you may find it difficult to see the person you love in discomfort or pain. You may feel redundant and unsure how best you can help, but be reassured that your presence is extremely useful.

In the early stages, offering words of support, massage (see page 286), drinks or food (if these are permitted) and just being there can be hugely helpful. You can try to help your partner to relax. She may like it if you can spray her face with a water spray or wipe it with a cool sponge. The other important part of your role is communicating with hospital staff on your partner's behalf and making sure that her birth plan (see page 128) is followed as much as it can be (bear in mind that although the birth plan needs to be respected, sometimes it cannot be followed exactly, so everyone concerned needs to be prepared to be flexible). You can also help your partner with any breathing exercises she has learnt and you may need to physically support her as she gets into position to give birth.

Once the baby arrives, you will be able to share your partner's delight, but it is important to be aware that newborn babies often look a little wrinkled and bloodied. You may be invited to cut the umbilical cord and then perhaps hold your baby skin-to-skin, which is important for the baby and will help the bonding process. If you don't feel an instant bond with your baby, or your partner doesn't seem to, don't worry as this isn't uncommon. It often takes time to absorb such a momentous event and to start to feel comfortable in one's new role.

What happens after the birth?

If the birth went smoothly and you and your baby are both fine, you may be discharged between four and six hours afterwards.

After ventouse or forceps
If you have had a ventouse or forceps delivery (see pages 302–3) or had stitches (see page 304) you are generally kept in hospital for at least one night. Your stitches will be checked before you go home to make sure they are healing properly, and you will be

given some general advice on how to keep the area clean and dry so that it continues to heal up quickly.

After a Caesarean

After a Caesarean section you will be monitored intensively for the first few hours to make sure that your blood pressure and pulse are normal and that you are not bleeding excessively. You will then be transferred to the postnatal ward, where you will be kept as mobile as possible. You will be given an injection of a drug to prevent the risk of deep-vein thrombosis. The catheter will be removed as soon as possible to reduce the chance of urinary tract infections. If you have had dissolvable stitches, these will not need to be removed, otherwise they will be taken out after five days. This should not prevent you going home as the community midwife can remove your stitches. These days, even after Caesarean section, you may go home within 48 hours if you are mobile, your wound is healing well and you have not bled excessively.

Checks before you go home

Before you go home your baby will be checked by the midwife or doctor to ensure that feeding is going well and that there are no other problems. The midwives will help you with breast-feeding and give you advice on clothing and bathing the baby too.

It is quite normal for you to bleed and this may continue for four to six weeks, decreasing gradually. Your midwife will make sure you are not bleeding excessively and that there are no signs of infections before you go home.

You will need some painkillers to take home, especially after a Caesarean section. It is important that you are passing urine well as a small number of women find this difficult after delivery and require a catheter for a few days. To make sure you do not get constipated it is important that you eat a healthy diet and drink plenty of water.

Pelvic floor exercise

If you have had a third-degree tear or difficult vaginal delivery the physiotherapist will see you to teach you pelvic floor exercises (see page 93). Try to do these as often and as early as possible as they will help reduce the risk of pelvic floor problems in the future.

15

The First Few Weeks
with Your Baby

Finding yourself at home with a new baby can be a daunting experience and you may not feel confident that you are doing things the right way to begin with. Your baby may seem so tiny and fragile, and it can be rather nerve-racking to feel that you are in sole charge of this delicate little person. However, feel reassured that most new parents go through the same worries and that it is always a steep learning curve to begin with. You may be feeling exhausted after the birth and if you've had a Caesarean section or stitches, you may be a little uncomfortable too. There will be a rush of hormones surging about in your body that may make your moods uneven, perhaps swinging from feeling tearful to elated in a short space of time.

Feeding your newborn

As a new mother you may not necessarily be sure how often and for how long you should be feeding your newborn baby. It always takes a bit of time to establish a feeding routine, so don't worry too much about this at the very beginning. Your midwife will have encouraged you to put your baby to your breast directly after he was born. Initially, you are producing colostrum (see page 172), which has very high levels of vitamins and protein as well as antibodies to help your baby fight off any infections, so it is important to do this even if you don't intend to breast-feed in the long-term.

Feeding little and often

At first, your baby will need to be fed frequently and for short spells, usually between eight and twelve times a day, although sometimes even more, depending on his size. It is important that you hold your baby in the right position for feeding and that he is properly latched on to your nipple. This helps you establish a good milk supply. Your midwife should be able to assist you with this. If you want to breast-feed but find that you are experiencing difficulties, or that it is causing you a great deal of discomfort or even pain, seek advice from a qualified breast-feeding counsellor. If you have had previous breast surgery or inverted nipples and are worried about breast-feeding, it may be helpful to talk to your midwife before you embark upon it. Many hospitals have breast-feeding counsellors, who can give useful tips and advice. There may also be advice on breast-feeding in your antenatal classes.

Although breast-feeding is undoubtedly the best and most natural way to feed your baby, for some mothers this isn't possible. If you are unable to breast-feed your baby, for whatever reason, don't let others make you feel guilty. The most important priority is your baby. Choose a first-stage formula milk (preferably organic), which is near in make-up to breast milk.

Don't try to implement a strict feeding schedule, or make your baby last for four hours between feeds, but feed him whenever he is hungry. If he is sleepy, wake him every three hours for a feed until he regains his birth weight. After that, you should be able to establish a pattern of approximately three hours between feeds during the day and four hours at night, as long as your baby is taking the required amount for his age and weight.

Limiting visitors

Although it is great that family and friends want to come and see your new baby, it can become rather overwhelming if your home is full of people all the time and particularly so if you are still feeling a little unconfident with your new baby. Try to make sure that you and your partner have the time you need to be with your baby by yourselves, so that you can learn how to deal with his needs. It can be hard to do this if you have a constant stream of well-meaning but overexcited visitors all trying to offer you their advice. This is a special time for you both to get to know your baby and you should not feel selfish about limiting visitors – this time for being with your newborn will never come round again.

Beware, too, of letting too many different people hold your baby. Babies are receptive to voices, touch and body language, so it is better for him if he has time to get used to his parents first and that they are meeting most of his needs in his early days. If your newborn is handed from one person to another a great deal, this can make him tired and fractious.

If a friend or relative has a cold or infection, suggest that they come to visit when they are better, so that you can avoid the risk of you or the baby becoming unwell, which is undesirable so early on.

Holding your baby

Cuddling your baby is an important part of the bonding process, and if you can do this calmly and with confidence, he is more likely to be calm and contented. When you pick your baby up, make sure you are close enough to do this comfortably. Bend over, slide your hand under his neck and spread your fingers out to support his head. Then slide your other hand between his legs. As you pick him up, straighten your back and move the hand supporting his head down his back until his head is in the crook of your arm. Then you will be able to move your supporting arm so that his bottom rests on your forearm, using your hand to hold his legs close to your body.

Nappy-changing

Most babies have their first bowel movement within 48 hours of being born. The nappy will be filled with meconium, which is a sticky black-green substance that was in the baby's intestines before he was born. As your baby gradually adjusts to life, his soiled nappies will vary in colour. If you are breast-feeding, the stools will probably look a bit like mustard, whereas a bottle-fed baby's stools are darker and thicker.

During the first few weeks, you will probably be changing your baby's nappy between eight and twelve times every day. If you make sure that you change him every time he has a bowel movement and before his nappy gets too wet, this will reduce the chances of him developing a red or irritated bottom, or developing nappy rash.

In the early days, wipe your baby's bottom with warm water and cotton wool rather than using baby wipes, which aren't always as gentle on a newborn baby's sensitive skin. If you are out and about and need to use wipes, buy perfume-free versions formulated for sensitive skin. There's no need to use baby powder as it clogs the skin and can get into his lungs.

Crying

All babies cry and it can be distressing for new parents, who may not be sure why their newborn seems 'upset'. There are a number of reasons newborn babies may be crying, and top of that list is hunger. If your new baby is fretful, it is a good idea to offer him a feed before you try anything else.

Tiredness

A common reason for babies to cry is tiredness. When they are under six weeks old, babies tend to get tired after about an hour of being awake. They may not be quite ready for sleep, but will need to be kept quiet and calm. Not all babies show obvious signs of tiredness, so in the early days, if he has been awake for an hour you could try taking him to a peaceful part of your home to wind down gently. If your baby under three months is awake for more than two hours at a time, he is likely to get overtired and he will find it more difficult to settle.

Wind

Another cause of crying can be wind. All babies take in a certain amount of air when they are feeding and most will bring it up again easily, but if you think wind could be a cause of your baby's crying, check that you are allowing sufficient time between feeds for him to digest his milk and take the time to wind him properly after each feed. Hold him carefully against your shoulder or in your lap while supporting his head under the chin and gently rub his back.

Getting back into shape

Your baby weight may not necessarily fall off easily – it takes us mere mortals a bit longer than it does the celebs, who are usually helped by personal trainers and nannies. Try not to get too disheartened and certainly don't worry about losing weight while you're breast-feeding. You'll probably lose some of your excess weight naturally, anyway. If, a few months down the line, you're still showing no signs of losing your baby weight, you might have to think about a sensible weight-loss diet. Don't be tempted to starve yourself and don't follow a 'fad' diet, because you'll find that you have reduced energy through lack of nutrients, and you may regain the weight afterwards just as quickly as you lost it.

If you are worried about gaining weight or not losing your baby weight, you can get dietary advice from your GP or follow a good-quality online slimming plan, which is ideal if you aren't able to get to slimming club meetings. If you are keen to go back to the gym ask the instructor about the best exercises to do to help firm up your pelvic floor. They can also advise you when the best time for starting sit-ups is.

When will we be ready to resume sex?

It is up to you as to when you start having sex after pregnancy and birth, but most GPs recommend waiting at least until after your six-week check-up, especially if you have had stitches. This advice applies to penetrative sex, so there is no reason why you should avoid other forms of intimacy.

Be aware that having a baby can have a big effect on you and your partner's libido, so be sure not to put any pressure on yourselves, keep the lines of communication open and just do what feels right, when it feels right.

Other things to be aware of

- If you are breast-feeding you will probably experience vaginal dryness, so it might be worth using a lubricant.

- Don't forget to use contraception if you don't want to get pregnant again so soon after the birth. Even if you are breast-feeding or your periods haven't yet resumed, a new pregnancy can still happen. Discuss your birth control options with your GP (some forms of the Pill aren't advisable if you are breast-feeding and some types of cap won't be suitable due to the way birth has affected your body). It's a good idea to stick to condoms until you have everything sorted out.

- If you've had an episiotomy or stitches be aware that you might experience some discomfort.

- Do your pelvic floor exercises (also known as Kegel exercises) to tone your pelvic floor after birth (see page 93). Imagine you need to pee and then try to stop yourself mid-stream. You should feel a tightening sensation. You can do these exercises throughout the day, especially at odd times such as when you are watching TV or waiting for the bus.

Tiredness and your sex life

Looking after a new baby can be exhausting, so it is not surprising that many new parents just don't feel in the mood for sex when their sleep is interrupted or limited. Relax and just accept that the first few months after your baby's birth are going to be a bit different from usual. If your libido still hasn't returned after a while and you are concerned about this, consult your GP.

Perception of your body

You may find that you think about your own body in a different way after your baby's birth to before it. You may feel that you were once a more sexual being than you are now. You feel changed and it can be hard to switch back from thinking about your breasts as a 'feeding station' to being a 'sensual being' (though, of course, breast-feeding can be a highly sensual experience). Your partner may be nervous about initiating sex or discover that he thinks about you differently now. All these feelings are common and natural. The best way to deal with anxieties is to talk about them and to have faith that, as time passes and you adapt to your new roles, you will find that your perception of yourself and your partner as sexual beings returns.

Coping with tiredness

No matter how many other mums warn you about tiredness and no matter how much you've read up on it, the reality is that the vast majority of new mums won't be prepared for the exhaustion they feel straight after their baby is born. As your body adapts to no longer being pregnant, the high levels of oestrogen, progesterone and endorphins that helped you through your pregnancy and labour dissipate, often leaving new mums with feelings of sadness and depression, known as the 'baby blues'. This, combined with the tiredness that comes with looking after a new baby, can feel overwhelming. But don't worry: these feelings are absolutely normal and you should soon feel better.

Make sure that you take care of yourself during this time. Mums often put others in front of themselves, but having a little bit of time to yourself each day to catch up on sleep or recharge your batteries doing something you enjoy will help to refresh you and make you more able to cope with the demands of a small baby. Don't think of it as being selfish – being happy and healthy is part of what makes a good mum. Keep up eating healthily and make sure that you sit down to eat, rather than eating standing up or on the go – it makes such a huge difference.

It's also a good idea to try to sleep when baby sleeps, even if that means napping in the middle of the day. It means that you can catch up on any sleep you miss during the night. If you're breast-feeding, it's a good idea to express some milk early in the day so that your partner can take charge of the late-night feeds, leaving you to wind down at the end of the day. This is ideal – you will get the chance to relax, and your partner will have some all-important bonding time with the baby.

Post-natal depression

It's absolutely normal to feel as if you're on an emotional roller coaster during the first few days after giving birth. However, some women feel overwhelmed by symptoms of depression such as sadness, guilt, fear, low self-esteem or anxiety. If you are having negative thoughts or experiencing persistent feelings such as the ones above, make sure you get help.

One in seven women suffer some form of post-natal depression in the three months after giving birth, so you mustn't feel guilty if you feel this way. It's a relatively common condition, and you are not alone – there are many people you can turn to for help. Your health visitor or GP will know what to do: post-natal depression is an illness, which is possible to treat with medication and with talking therapies, such as Cognitive Behavioural Therapy. Make sure to talk to your partner, family and friends and let them know how you are feeing. Perhaps there are things that they can do to take the pressure off you. Do not feel as if you are weak by asking for help – we all need assistance at various times in our lives, and ultimately you are making sure of your baby's well-being by getting the help that you need.

Getting your baby into a routine

You may well find that getting your baby into a good routine makes life run a lot more smoothly for you and your family. A routine that runs from 7 am to 7 pm usually works best for young babies as it fits in with their natural sleeping rhythms and their need to feed little and often. It's a good idea to try to achieve a regular sleeping pattern, where your baby settles well in the evening, feeds and settles at around 10.30pm, then only wakes once in the night for a feed and goes back to sleep quickly until 6–7am.

An early pattern

Establishing a regular routine or daily pattern early on in his life can be hugely beneficial for your baby, and will also help you to feel more confident about being able to meet his needs. By following this advice, you will find that he settles more quickly and is more contented. If you continue to keep the routine going, you may find that he cries less and is calmer, which will allow you to have more time to yourself.

- Try not to let your baby sleep for very long stretches between feeds during the day, as this will mean that he is more likely to be hungry during the night and will wake up wanting to be fed.

- If you wake your baby every three hours during the early days and offer him a feed, he will be more likely to sleep for a longer stretch at night (the three hours being from the beginning of one feed to the beginning of the next).

- In order to ensure that he sleeps his longer stretch between 11pm and 6–7am, he will need to sleep well during the evening.

- Resist the temptation to try to keep your baby awake during the evening. You may think that doing this will mean he is more likely to sleep at night because he will be 'more tired'. In fact, the opposite is often the case as babies can become fretful and irritable, needing frequent feeding during the evening. They then take only a small feed at 10pm and wake up hungry a couple of hours later.

● Breast milk is produced on a supply-and-demand basis (the more the baby feeds the more milk is produced), and demand feeding can lead to a pattern of feeding every couple of hours, which is likely to be exhausting.

● If your baby's daytime sleep and feeds have been planned around a structure and he feeds at 6pm, followed by a sleep between 7pm and 10pm, he will wake up ready for a full feed then, which will help him to go to sleep for longer during the night.

As a new parent, you will find that there is much to learn in the weeks and months ahead. Getting to know your baby and caring for him isn't always easy, but it is certainly one of life's most rewarding experiences.

Conclusion

Congratulations! You have completed your pregnancy journey and now have a lovely little baby in your arms! These first few days can be such a joy as you rediscover the world through the eyes of your new baby.

There will be many firsts in the months and years to come – baby's first smile, his first words, his first steps. It's a wonderful time of discovery and exploration for parents and baby alike, and it may feel as if it's over all too soon! This period of time is a wonderful one to cherish.

While countless numbers of women have had babies, and it's fantastic to be able to draw on their experience and advice, each baby, each new mum and dad, are unique and special. You might have finished your pregnancy journey but you're about to embark on another, even more challenging one. But the journey will be rewarding too as each new milestone passes and your baby grows into a toddler, child and adult. Welcome to the world of parenthood – it's an exciting and ever-changing place to be.

Resources

Healthcare

NHS
Clinical information and health advice.
www.nhs.uk; www.nhsdirect.nhs.uk
0845 4647

Healthy Start
Information on nutrition, plus details for applying for Healthy Start food vouchers.
www.healthystart.nhs.uk

Support groups

National Childbirth Trust (NCT)
The leading charity offering information and support for pregnancy, birth and early parenthood. They offer antenatal, postnatal and parenting courses across the UK.
www.nct.org.uk

Sure Start Children's Centres
Early learning and daycare services for children under five.
www.direct.gov.uk

Childminding

The National Childminding Association (NCMA)
Guidance on choosing childcare.
www.ncma.org.uk

Maternity leave and benefits and child tax credits

HMRC
Information on child tax credits.
www.hmrc.gov.uk

Department of Work and Pensions
Information on statutory maternity pay (SMP).
www.dwp.gov.uk

Directgov
Information on maternity leave and pay. Includes downloadable claim forms for maternity allowance and Sure Start maternity grants.
www.direct.gov.uk

Job Centre
Maternity allowance information.
Jobcentre Plus
0800 055 6688

Citizens Advice Bureau
Information on maternity leave and pay.
www.citizensadvice.org.uk

Miscarriage and ectopic pregnancy

The Ectopic Pregnancy Trust

Information, education and support for those affected by ectopic pregnancies and the health professionals who care for them.

www.ectopic.org.uk

020 7733 2653

The Miscarriage Association

Information and support for anyone affected by the loss of a baby in pregnancy.

www.miscarriageassociation.org.uk

01924 200 799

Sands

Support for anyone affected by the death of a baby.

www.uk-sands.org

020 7436 5881

Emotional and mental health issues

The National Childbirth Trust helpline

Practical and emotional support in all areas of pregnancy, birth and early parenthood.

www.nct.org.uk

0300 330 0700

Mind
Advice and support for anyone with mental health concerns. Includes information on postnatal depression.
www.mind.org.uk
0845 766 0163

The Samaritans
24-hour support for anyone experiencing feelings of distress or despair.
www.samaritans.org
08457 909 090

Relationship advice

Relate
The UK's largest provider of relationship support, offering advice, counselling, workshops and therapy.
www.relate.org.uk
0300 100 1234

Problems with addiction or abuse

Alcoholics Anonymous
Support for alcoholics.
www.alcoholics-anonymous.org.uk
0845 769 7555

Ad-fam
Support for families affected by drugs and alcohol.
www.adfam.org.uk

Drink Line

A 24-hour confidential helpline for alcoholics or their friends or families.
0800 917 8282

The National Domestic Violence helpline

Confidential helpline on domestic violence, open 24 hours a day.
www.nationaldomesticviolencehelpline.org.uk
0808 2000 247

Women's Aid

Domestic and sexual violence support, with a free 24-hour national helpline.
www.womensaid.org.uk
0808 2000 247

Women's Refuge

Assistance for women suffering from domestic violence, with a free 24-hour national helpline.
refuge.org.uk
0808 2000 247

Useful baby equipment

SnoozeShade

Sun and sleep shades that help babies nap on-the-go. Give Baby protection from sun, wind, chill and light rain.
www.snoozeshade.com
01932 500 427

Contented Baby Newsletter

To learn more about Gina Ford's books, visit Gina's official websites at www.contentedbaby.com and www.contentedtoddler.com and sign up to receive Gina's free monthly newsletter, which is full of useful information, tips and advice as well as answers to questions about parenting issues and even a recipe or two.

You may also want to take the opportunity to become part of Gina's online community by joining one or both of the websites. As a member you'll receive a monthly online magazine with a personal message from Gina, along with a selection of the latest exclusive features on topical issues from guest contributors and members. You'll be able to access more than 2,000 frequently asked questions about feeding, sleeping and development answered by Gina and her team, as well as many case histories not featured in the Contented Little Baby series of books.

www.contentedbaby.com; www.contentedtoddler.com
www.contentedbaby.com/shop-directory.htm

Contented Baby Consultation Service

Gina offers a one-to-one personal telephone consultation service for parents who wish for specialist help in establishing healthy feeding and sleeping habits, as laid out in the Contented Baby and Toddler routine books. If you would like further details of how a personal consultation with Gina works, we would request that in the first instance you send a detailed feeding and sleeping diary for 48 hours, along with a concise summary of what you think your problem is, using the contact form on www.contentedbaby.com.

Acknowledgements

I would like to express my gratitude to all the parents I have worked with over the years. Their feedback has been an enormous help in writing my books. I would also like to thank my publisher Fiona MacIntyre and editor Louise Francis for their constant encouragement and faith in my work, and thanks to the rest of the team at Vermilion for all their hard work on the book. Thank you to my co-author, consultant obstetrician Charlotte Chaliha, for her fantastic work on the book. She has done such a great job of explaining complex medical matters in a clear and accessible format, and has been a real pleasure to work with.

A special thank you to my agent Emma Kirby, for her continued dedication and support, and to Kate Brian and Laura Simmons, for their efforts in gathering information for the book. Thank you to Alison Jermyn, Jane Waygood, Peter Ritchie and Rory Jenkins, and the rest of the team at Contentedbaby.com, for their support while I was writing this book and their wonderful work on the website.

And, finally, I am ever grateful for the huge support I receive from the thousands of readers of my books who take the time to contact me – a huge thank you to you all and much love to your contented babies.

Gina Ford

Index

H. 1/15

The Contented Pregnancy